Charcot in Morocco

Charcot in Morocco

Introduction, notes and
translation by Toby Gelfand

University of Ottawa Press
Ottawa

uOttawa

© University of Ottawa Press, 2012

The University of Ottawa Press acknowledges with gratitude the support extended to its publishing list by Heritage Canada through its Book Publishing Industry Development Program, by the Canada Council for the Arts, by the Canadian Federation for the Humanities and Social Sciences through its Award to Scholarly Publications Program, by the Social Sciences and Humanities Research Council, and by the University of Ottawa.

LIBRARY AND ARCHIVES CANADA CATALOGUING IN PUBLICATION

Charcot, J. M. (Jean Martin), 1825–1893
Charcot in Morocco / introduction, notes and translation
by Toby Gelfand.

Translated from the French.
Includes bibliographical references.
Issued also in electronic format.
ISBN 978-0-7766-0774-0

1. Charcot, J. M. (Jean Martin), 1825–1893--Travel--Morocco.
2. Morocco--Description and travel.
3. Tétouan (Morocco)--Description and travel.
4. Nervous system--Diseases. 5. Jews--Diseases--Morocco--Tétouan.
I. Gelfand, Toby, 1942- II. Title.

DT309.C5313 2012   916.4'043   C2012-900728-5

To Michel Bonduelle, friend and colleague

Table of Contents

Preface and Acknowledgments

Charcot remains an enigmatic figure. This despite a large body of scientific work *by* him, amounting to some fourteen substantial volumes, and a much more voluminous literature *about* him. These provide the reader with a good understanding of the pioneer of neurology but are much less successful with respect to Charcot the man. The same can be said about the outpouring of contemporary tributes by devoted students following Charcot's sudden death in 1893. Sigmund Freud and Pierre Janet, both on their way to becoming masters of psychology, each contributed insightful appreciations of their teacher, but neither captured his elusive personality. Others, who knew Charcot better, wrote longer eulogies with more personal details without achieving the "intimate" portrait that they invoked. After all, these were eulogists, admirers, for the most part, of the deceased.

Beyond the obvious issue of bias in the eyewitness sources lies a more fundamental deficiency—a paucity of the kinds of autobiographical sources upon which biographers depend. Charcot's correspondence is scattered around the world, much of it undoubtedly lost, the rest unpublished or, at best, published in fragments. As I explain in my introduction, the personal day book he kept during his Moroccan voyage of 1887 offers the reader a rare glimpse of Charcot *par lui-même*. Here we find unselfconsciously on display Charcot's inner monologue as the famous French physician experiences the "Orient."

This project owes its origins to the generosity of the late R. Allart-Charcot, the grandson by marriage of Jean-Martin Charcot. In 1986 Monsieur Allart-Charcot provided me with a photocopy of his grandfather-in-law's century-old journal. He and his wife welcomed me repeatedly into their home in

Neuilly-sur-Seine, a hospitality continued by their daughter and her husband, the Vallin-Charcots, with whom I had the pleasure and privilege to reside for several days in December 1996. There I was able to immerse myself in family papers relating to the Moroccan voyage, including the original drawings by Charcot, which appear in the illustrations to this book. Along with many other scholars, I am grateful to these family descendants, whose keen appreciation of *patrimoine* has preserved and maintained what was originally the neurologist's country retreat on a *rez-de-chaussé* housing a treasure of personal correspondence, albums, books, art, craft and woodwork, and sculpture.

I thank Mme Véronique Leroux-Hugon, conservateur of the Bibliothèque Charcot at the Salpêtrière hospital. Her intimate knowledge of and unflagging dedication to this unique repository have been a precious resource during annual research visits beginning in the mid-1980s. Without her expert guidance and cataloguing skills, Charcot's vast original nineteenth-century library and his boxes of manuscripts would present an unnavigable labyrinth to scholars.

I especially thank two physicians, Michel Bonduelle and the late Georges Sée. Both men, *anciens internes des hôpitaux de Paris* from the early decades of the twentieth century when that title carried an elite cachet, kindly and painstakingly aided me in deciphering Charcot's handwritten journal. Needless to say, all shortcomings are my own responsibility.

Closer to home, my bilingual and technologically fluent administrative assistant, Chanel Ghazzawi, has patiently and with much appreciated good humor about French accent marks, helped with finishing touches to the transcription and translation of the manuscript. Last, but far from least, I thank my wife, Deborah Gorham, for her perceptive advice based on generous readings and re-readings.

I

Introduction

1.1 *A physician at the pinnacle of fame: 1887*

By the mid-1880s, Jean-Martin Charcot (1825–1893) had become the leading authority in France and, arguably, in the world, on diseases of the nervous system. "People had come to realize," Sigmund Freud wrote of his French mentor, "that the activities of this man were a part of the assets of the nation's 'gloire.'"[1] In 1887, when he embarked for a summer holiday vacation that would culminate in Morocco, Charcot's reputation within and beyond medical circles had reached a pinnacle, undimmed by the skepticism that emerged subsequently and that even tinged Freud's otherwise admiring funeral eulogy.[2]

Born in Paris into a middle-class artisan family, Charcot based his knowledge and immense reputation on a long career at the hospice of the Salpêtrière, the city's centuries-old mental asylum and refuge for chronically ill and elderly women.[3] There he worked during his final year as a hospital intern in 1852, doing research that resulted in an important thesis for his medical degree on gout and chronic joint disease. Ten years later, Charcot returned to the Salpêtrière to be its chief physician for the remaining thirty years of his life. Here he made a series of fundamental contributions to the understanding of diseases of the nervous system, several of which would bear his name and, taken together, made that name synonymous with leadership of the "school of the Salpêtrière" and the emergence of neurology as a distinct medical specialty. Whatever titles of success Charcot achieved, and there were many, notably his election to the elite French Academy of Sciences in 1883, flowed, as he recognized at a banquet celebrating that triumph, from his power base at "that good old Salpêtrière hospice."[4]

In the early 1880s, Charcot acquired, with the backing of the Gambetta government and despite the reticence of his colleagues on the Paris Faculty of Medicine, a clinical professorship, created especially for him, in diseases of the nervous system. The new professorial chair served as the centerpiece to a multi-faceted research and teaching institute at the Salpêtrière, unrivalled in the world, with associated staff and laboratories of histopathology, ophthalmology and otology, electrotherapy, photography, an art studio, and a museum.

Charcot's lectures and demonstrations drew a large lay as well as a medical professional audience, numbering in the hundreds, to dramatic public lessons in the hospital amphitheater. Here he presented, literally on stage, patients illustrating the entire spectrum of diseases of the nervous system. But most commonly selected for demonstration and appreciated by viewers were flamboyant cases of hysteria in women and the more novel male counterpart of the same ailment. One journalist, fascinated as well as horrified by the spectacle of male and partially clad female patients, subjected like "automatons," to the will of the demonstrator/hypnotist, entitled the account of the public lesson he witnessed in May 1885, "The century of Charcot":

> This century will be the century of nervous diseases in two respects. First because they determine and control all actions; second, because they will have been studied so profoundly that the secrets of their evil will be revealed. That is why it will perhaps not be the century of Victor Hugo, nor the century of Napoleon, but rather the century of Charcot.[5]

Leçons du mardi, or Tuesday lessons, less rehearsed than the public spectacles and open only to a select group of students and invited witnesses, began in the early 1880s at the Salpêtrière's newly-built out-patient clinic. Again, patients with hysteria predominated with its panoply of symptoms—paralyses and contractures, sensory deficits including impairment of vision, hearing, and speech, and the full-fledged convulsive attacks of hystero-epilepsy or *grande hystérie*, whose four phases Charcot had defined. These symptoms, when not already displayed, would be elicited "experimentally" by hypnosis, a technique Charcot had rehabilitated in presentations to the Academy of Sciences in the late 1870s.

Such demonstrations made Charcot famous beyond medical circles. Fittingly, he chose an action scene of an hysteric being hypnotized for a large group portrait of himself and his entourage gathered about a beautiful décolleté Blanche Wittmann, a well-known patient on the threshold of an attack of hystero-epilepsy. The canvas, by André Bouillet, titled simply *Une leçon clinique à la Salpêtrière*, drew crowds and received admiring reviews in the press at the Paris spring salon of 1887 [**fig. 1**]. By this time, the neurologist had become a celebrity, his striking profile often likened to that of Napoleon [**fig. 2**], intentionally cultivated according to some, and a persona of symbolic stature in the writings of Guy de Maupassant, Tolstoy, and their lesser contemporaries.[6]

If the exotic and eroticized image of hysteria came to dominate Charcot's public persona, the neurologist firmly advocated positivist clinical and anatomical investigation of an ailment he believed was physiological and ultimately would be traced to disordered functioning of the higher nervous centers in the cerebral cortex. Since hysteria, was deemed to be a "mimic" capable of taking on the form of other diseases, Charcot routinely cautioned physicians to suspect its presence before diagnosing more grave and much less prevalent ailments of the nervous system.

Charcot's fame drew extraordinary numbers of patients, students, and colleagues to his hospital clinic and to his private consultation rooms in his sumptuous mansion at 217 Boulevard Saint Germain. Clients spanned the social spectrum from royalty, like the Emperor of Brazil, to homeless vagrants, typified by so-called wandering Jews from as far away as Russia, Central Asia, and the Middle East.

Among fellow physicians and medical students attracted to the Salpêtrière school, British, Germans and Austrians, Americans, and Russians predominated, but they also came from more remote corners of the globe. Autographed expressions of gratitude to "*le maître*" appear on the hundreds of reprints of their publications sent to Paris and bound into volumes in his library. One visiting Japanese student, Kinnosuke Miura, promised to seek to put into practice what he had learned when he returned to Tokyo.[7] Another young neuropathologist, Sigmund Freud of Vienna, had a similar transformative experience when he came to Paris in October 1885 to spend more than four months at the Salpêtrière, where he too fell under Charcot's spell. Traveling toward Charcot was a well-traveled route and a familiar story.

1.2 *A traveler himself*

Charcot personally loved to travel abroad and did so as often as possible. Throughout a medical career that spanned most of the second half of the nineteenth century, the physician's reasons for setting forth ranged from business to pleasure. He usually managed to combine both as his summer excursions became annual events from the late 1870s until literally his final days.[8]

At the outset of his career, shortly after receiving his Paris medical degree in 1853, the young doctor accompanied a wealthy patient, the banker Benoit Fould, on a several-month excursion through Italy. Forty years later in the midst of a holiday tour of Bourgogne with two younger colleagues, heart failure brought a sudden end to Charcot's life. Indeed the fact that the still active nearly sixty-eight-year-old physician had this time restricted his voyage within Northern France indicated a faltering health. In earlier years, Charcot seldom failed to venture throughout most of Europe and, occasionally, beyond its borders.

He made many visits to Great Britain before, during, and after the War of 1870–71, mainly for the purpose of attending professional meetings, but also to see personal friends in London, where his family had taken refuge during the war. On his final visit, just a few months before his death, Charcot crossed the Channel as a member of an official commission sent to examine the medical status of an accused criminal in exile.[9] On two occasions he made the long railway journey to Russia, the first time in 1881 and again a decade later, accompanied by his two children. The trips to Russia came in response to wealthy patients' requests for his medical services, but they also involved visiting colleagues and local medical institutions and being the guest of honor at lavish banquets. After France's disastrous defeat by Prussia in 1870, Charcot refused to set foot in the new German Empire, but he continued to visit Northern and Central Europe. High-profile trips, such as those to Russia and to the International Medical Congress of 1881 in London, where Charcot's prestige in the French delegation rivaled that of Louis Pasteur, received considerable notice in the popular as well as in the medical press.[10]

When he ventured south to the French Midi, to Italy and Spain, Charcot tended to favor personal pleasure over professional duty. But he found it difficult to draw a sharp distinction between work and recreation. The proverbial "busman on holiday," the physician could not pass a church or museum without examining art works and artifacts for what they might reveal of the history of disease, a pastime he eventually transformed into professional publications.[11] With his reputation preceding him, Charcot was often obliged to grant consultations to importuning patients and colleagues.[12]

1.3 *Voyage to Morocco*

Thus, in July 1887, at the height of his fame and with a lifetime of travel experience, Charcot set out once again for Spain. Of all his annual summer holiday travels, this voyage culminating with seven days in Morocco would be his most ambitious adventure and his first personal exposure to North Africa.[13] The Moroccan portion of the trip resulted in Charcot's richest travel account by far: a day book, running to ninety-five manuscript pages (nearly 14,000 words) [**fig. 4**], the detailed description evidencing the special interest the diarist attached to this excursion.[14]

According to his own headings, the contents of Charcot's journal are as follows:

1st day. From Algeciras to Ceuta (**Ms A fol. 1-a**).
2nd day. The fishery and the frontier of Morocco—the penal colony (**2-c**).
3rd day. From Ceuta to Tetuan. The Moor's House (**Ms B 3-a**).
4th day. The Jewish wedding—the Jewish quarter—the market—the town—Moorish houses (**Ms A 5-c**).
5th day. Jew's house. Consultations. School (**10-c**).
6th day. [from Tetuan to Ceuta] [August 13] (**13-c**).

No similar personal journal exists for Charcot's many other voyages. For those the main source is the correspondence that the physician dutifully posted to his wife, who almost always remained at home. The husband's letters contain sketches of places and persons to which Charcot added written comments, usually brief captions, but sometimes fuller descriptions for the more elaborate drawings to be kept in albums of his travels. None of this material bears comparison with the detailed narrative of the Moroccan visit.

Charcot's Moroccan journal is a unique document for him (and the historian) in several respects: in its sheer length and detail but also in the intimate, relaxed, colorful, at times frankly exuberant quality of a first-person narrative written primarily for oneself, even if it were later to be shared with family and friends. The journal offers rare access to an otherwise elusive figure who said little of a spontaneous nature in public. The neurologist preferred to work behind the scenes, letting subordinates speak, and, more often, publish on his behalf. Charcot's publications consisted almost entirely of carefully prepared lectures gathered and edited by his hospital assistants and interns in which *"Monsieur Charcot,"* thus filtered, addresses the reader. Even the more intimate and informal *Leçons du Mardi,* two volumes of putative transcripts of clinical dialogues between Charcot and patients who came to the Salpêtrière out-patient clinic at the end of the 1880s, were less spontaneous than they purported to be. A notable and highly unusual medical text, which appears to provide a literal replication in conversational style of what transpired during the clinical examination, the *Leçons du Mardi* were in fact carefully planned in advance with selected patients and then edited for publication.[15]

Historians, following most contemporary accounts, tend to portray Charcot as an authoritarian and rather austere medical leader, a *"grand patron"* who was at once intimidating and shy, if not secretive. The Moroccan journal reveals a less pretentious figure possessed of a rough and ready sense of humor, someone who did not always take himself or others so seriously. The eagerness with which the famous physician proceeded across the torrid open square in Tetuan, leaving his colleagues, to see a charlatan perform, for example, appears in stark contrast with the austere professor surrounded by his acolytes whom Parisians flocked to see at the Salpêtrière.[16]

The journal appears to have been written at intervals during the voyage. One wonders when Charcot would have found the time given the full days that typically began at daybreak. The diarist makes no reference to writing in retrospect, or indeed to the act of writing. He consistently employs the present tense, except for very few mentions of something that happened the previous day or that would take place a day or two later, indicating a brief delay at times in composition. This form of writing conveys the impression that the events are transpiring in real time.

Charcot thus seems to have jotted down his Moroccan journal in bursts, with scant attention, if any, to style, none to revision, and no thought of publishing this personal record. There are few alterations in the manuscript, such as crossing out or insertion of words, or marginalia. The punctuation is careless, often lacking capital letters which makes it at times difficult to tell where one sentence ends and another begins. French accent marks are frequently omitted. Charcot's handwriting is firm, and recognizably similar to that in his letters and other manuscripts, but, as might be expected from what has already been said about its manner of composition, the text is sometimes difficult to decipher resulting in a number of illegible words. Minor errors and gaps suggest that the manuscript probably was not reread by the author.

In addition to the Moroccan journal, and supplementing its account, Charcot wrote several letters during the trip to Madame Charcot. So did their daughter, Jeanne, and their son, Jean, who both accompanied their father on this voyage as they had often done in the past [**fig. 3**].[17]

Charcot's record of his Moroccan voyage may be usefully compared with the recently discovered and now-published *Souvenirs sur le Maroc* by Eugene Delacroix, a narrative that the artist composed and carefully reworked with the intention of publication some ten or twelve years after his visit to Morocco.[18] Delacroix's voyage of 1832 served as a well-known precedent for French travelers, including Charcot, to that part of colonial North Africa. One obvious feature that the physician's journal shared with the artist's travel notebooks was their recourse to pictorial sketches [*croquis*] to supplement the verbal account. This was a common practice and one that Charcot, himself a competent artist, employed regularly in his letters as well as in his medical publications.[19] Unlike the artist's superb drawings and watercolors during his six-month visit to Morocco, Charcot, with the exception of a few watercolors, confined himself during a brief voyage of just one week to simple ink sketches rather than attempting more ambitious depictions.

Charcot's preparatory notes for his trip show that he had Delacroix in mind. Thanks to his friend and traveling companion, the art critic Philippe Burty (1830–1890), an expert on Delacroix, the physician had ready access to the artist's unpublished Moroccan *cahiers*, consisting of journal and drawings. In particular, Charcot jotted down references to Delacroix's account of the Jewish wedding he had witnessed in Tangier on 21 February 1832 (and painted in a celebrated masterpiece several years later) along with the artist's various uses of color.[20] Charcot would cite the precedent of Delacroix when he attended a Jewish wedding on his own trip.[21] Ironically, Burty, alarmed by the prospect of sea sickness, remained behind when the group crossed the straits of Gibraltar to North Africa.

For Charcot, Morocco represented an exciting prospect, a glimpse of what he called "Africa" but perceived as the Moorish Orient. "My little expedition,"[22] as he later modestly referred to the brief excursion, presented at the time a relished opportunity for the clinician to turn his considerable powers of observation to novel and, for him, exotic sights and customs: "Employing a searching gaze [*œil scrutateur*], we look into everything open to us."[23] His comments reveal as much, perhaps more, about the observer than the observed. On the epistemological level, Charcot naively assumed that his own presence did not affect the subjects of his gaze. Thus, traversing the Jewish quarter of Tetuan, he remarks, "Nothing detracts from the picture [*le tableau*] except us, and we don't look at ourselves. . . . Our passing through caused no stir anywhere."[24]

Charcot's assumption of pure or unmediated objective observation also pervaded his clinical interpretation of hysteria and hypnotism at the Salpêtrière. Contemporary critics pointed out that neurologist's unbounded confidence in the validity of his observations and interventions was unwarranted, citing the distorting effects of suggestion on the part of the investigator and "expectant attention" or unconscious compliance by patients. But the neurologist gave little credence to such objections, and he flatly rejected the possibility that patients might be able to mislead him unintentionally or by outright deception.

Despite touches of humor and ironic reflections, Charcot brought a serious and conscientious approach to the task of being a tourist. The itinerary he chose was to be followed scrupulously by the group. Inconveniences, notably the intense heat of the summer season in North Africa, were to be stoically endured: "we are not here to amuse ourselves. Putting up with all the vermin in creation is part of the program,"[25] he wrote, as the travel party suffered in a wretched inn in the port town of Ceuta. Charcot's exuberance sometimes broke through, as on the return trip by sea from Tetuan to Ceuta when the physician boyishly likened their boat's retreat from a storm into a cove to a maneuver worthy of the Barbary pirates of old, "ready to do some dastardly deed."[26] The traveler ate heartily, amazing his hosts "with our insatiable appetite . . . never have they seen so many meals and such copious meals prepared! For sure, this kind of cure by means of exercise in the open air at an average temperature of 35 degrees in the shade is something to be recommended."[27] He did not, however, care for Arab cuisine: "no Arab meats, no *kouskousou*, but good Spanish food" **(A, 9-d)**. He expressed similar European preferences with regard to the local musicians in the group hired to play for them. After trying in vain to follow the unfamiliar melody, the tired physician slipped away "stealthily" to bed **(A, 10-a–10-c)**.[28]

As for reflections on sexuality, there is literally nothing more than a fleeting glimpse by the man whom Freud credited with an insight into the sexual origins of hysteria.[29] On entering a room of women in a well-to-do Muslim household to which they had been invited, Charcot remarked:

> A flurry of emotion, doubtless feigned, a pretended surprise ensued when we entered. A lady of mature years, who appeared beautiful to me, quickly fled, but not before showing us her face. That left 4 or 5 negresses, who shamelessly stayed where they were. Moreover, they were very beautiful, their arms and legs nude, their bodies lightly clothed in a clear fabric. They certainly do not belong to the religion whose acolytes cover up. **(A, 8-d)**

The Moroccan journal begins on Monday, August 8, 1887 with the crossing of the straits of Gibraltar from Algeciras in Spain to Ceuta on the North African coast. The group had departed Paris on July 18 and had pursued the following itinerary: Madrid (July 26), Cordova (July 30), Seville (August 1), Cadiz (August 4), Algeciras (August 5). They would return from Morocco via Malaga, Granada, and Saint Sebastien to arrive back in Paris on August 29.[30]

Charcot immediately heightens the sense of risky adventure by dwelling on the potential hazards of the sea crossing. It was here that Philippe Burty, frightened by the prospect and, it appears, by the warnings of another member of the group, probably the writer Paul Arène,[31] chose to remain behind.

1.4 *Tetuan:* "une perle, un bijou"[32]

The ultimate destination of the Charcot travel party was Tetuan, a town of about twenty-five thousand inhabitants located approximately forty kilometers to the south of Ceuta. Tetuan's population consisted, in Charcot's words, of a majority of "*arabes de toute sorte*," estimated at around sixteen thousand, and about four thousand Jews. There were also black Moroccans and very few Europeans. Charcot wrote to his wife that there were probably not even twenty Spaniards in Tetuan compared with twenty thousand in Tangiers.[33] Tracing its origins to the settlement at the end of the fifteenth century by Andalusian Moors who built the walled town, Tetuan was known for its picturesque setting on a sloping valley between mountains and sea, for its exquisitely decorated wealthy Moorish houses, for a tile works, and for a reputation as a former haven for Barbary pirates. A Spanish military expedition captured the town amid much destruction in 1860 but withdrew after a treaty that extracted a heavy indemnity from the Moroccans. Thus, in 1887, Tetuan remained part of the kingdom of Morocco, in contrast to Ceuta and its immediate environs, which were Spanish possessions.

Obviously delighted to have escaped the familiar trappings of European civilization, Charcot reveled in what he perceived as the authenticity of "a genuine Arab town, the likes of which cannot be seen in Algeria or Tunis. It's pristine, really pristine."[34] He was probably not far off in this assessment. Aside from the coastal Spanish possessions, Morocco remained more pristine than its North African neighbors or, as another French visitor at about the same time remarked, less modified by European intrusion than just about anywhere else colonial empires had ventured, including India or China.[35] Lacking telegraphic communication, rail lines, or roads, the interior of Morocco remained difficult to access for those not on official business or having the wealth and energy to provide for their own protection. While Delacroix's extensive voyage came as a traveling companion of Count Charles de Mornay, special ambassador heading a French diplomatic mission to the Emperor of Morocco, Charcot's brief excursion, neither official nor equipped for long distances, did not extend into the interior of the kingdom.[36] Nevertheless, in 1887, the overland route to Tetuan demanded, as Charcot described it, a lengthy and difficult day's journey.[37] Thanks to Charcot's influential contacts ("I am introduced as someone who is a personage"),[38] he was able to recruit considerable assistance. The travel party was met by the director of the penal colony upon arrival at Ceuta, provided with guides, servants, and supplies, and permitted to use the newly installed military telegraph. In Tetuan, the Spanish consul and members of his embassy welcomed and escorted their French visitors.

In a manner characteristic of tourists, Charcot sought out the exotic with delight, while he expressed disappointment at the few reminders of European presence. Coming across a discarded recent copy of his least favorite newspaper, *Le Figaro*, in the midst of the desert during their day-long trek from Ceuta to Tetuan was a striking instance of sudden disillusionment that Charcot presents in an amusing light for the reader:

> Here we are, far from Europe, from France, from Paris
> . . . here there's nothing commonplace . . . places nearly
> unexplored. I was enjoying the sensation imparted by the
> idea 'of an unknown well where one is the first to drink'
> as Lucretius says. Alas a piece of yellowed newspaper lies
> on the ground. It seems to have been used to hold some
> food, unless it was for something else . . . I read in large
> letters, *Le Figaro*!!![39]

There were other discordant sights: "Sometimes a few of those big brilliant silver balls with which the bourgeoisie in our country, who lack taste, decorate our gardens."[40] Mirrors and clocks, seemingly from Paris shops, spoiled the decor of Moorish interiors; the Jewish bridegroom wore a European suit and melon top hat. In criticizing such dissonance, Charcot, at the same time, showed a sense of cultural relativity when he noted that Parisians collect foreign bibelots in a similar spirit.[41] The physician's display of his personal discriminating artistic judgment casts doubt on Edmond de Goncourt's haughty dismissal of Charcot and his family as tasteless bourgeois.[42]

The Charcot travel party reached Tetuan on the evening of Monday, August 9th after a thirteen-hour trek begun at dawn from Ceuta [**figs. 5, 6, and 7**]. He and his daughter rode on mules ("where I arrange myself like someone disabled . . . which I am . . . Jeanne only has infirmities which are natural to her sex")[43] while the other visitors, guides, bodyguards, and a Negro servant walked. Charcot's vivid account of this traverse speaks for itself **(B, 6-10)**.[44] Worth noting, however, is the rare instance where he betrays a sign of losing control, fearing that they may have wandered astray after some six hours of walking. Rather than express anxiety or fear directly, Charcot notes his anger toward the guides: "We begin to berate the Moors of the Emperor who led us down this wrong path."[45]

The arrival in Tetuan after dark when the city gates had been closed also produced some tense moments. Eventually, the gate-keeper, whom Charcot could not understand but whom he imagined to be hurling insults ("Christian dogs . . . go sleep in the open air"),[46] was persuaded to let the travelers enter the town. Until then, Charcot's prestige had ensured a welcoming reception. Furnished with letters from the Spanish authorities, the travel party had been cordially received by a large delegation at the port of Ceuta. Charcot, ever ready with a literary metaphor, described their leader: "tall, thin, very helpful, wearing an absurd cravat and an endlessly long white jacket which nicely throws into relief his Don Quixote-like form" **(A, 1-d)**.[47] This was the prison director who immediately ordered the menacing-looking surrounding persons ["*hommes de mine assez sinistre*"], a group of convicts from the galleys, to carry the arrivals' luggage to their inn. The following day the French party was taken on a tour first of the prison and then of a large fishing establishment. Charcot, a confirmed lover of animals, pitied the fish, "these poor creatures,"[48] as they struggled in vain to escape the nets.

In Tetuan the group settled at the fonda Espagnole **[fig. 8]**, a comfortable lodging that they found much superior to the inn at Ceuta. The following morning the Charcot entourage embarked on a full schedule of sightseeing despite withering temperatures that they estimated to be in excess of forty degrees centigrade. At Ceuta, crowds had already stared at them, calling them either madmen or "Englishmen" ("Ingles") to have visited at the hottest time of the year. And yet Charcot, at nearly sixty-two years of age, corpulent, his legs stiffened to the point of rigidity, in his own opinion "handicapped" ["*infirme*"], had accomplished the overland journey without apparent difficulty or complaint. The intense heat did not keep him from his itinerary over the next three days in Tetuan. "Papa astonishes me," Jeanne Charcot wrote to her mother the morning after their long journey overland,

> He gets in and out of the boat, up and down from the mule. Thirteen hours en route and he can still be ready to go out half-past six in the morning![49]

1.5 *The Jewish Wedding*

Charcot's written and pictorial account of Tetuan ranged over the inhabitants, their housing, food and drink, dress, architecture, art and music, marriage and burial ceremonies, and a few medical observations. He devoted his longest and most detailed description to a Jewish wedding he attended on the first morning in Tetuan. "The following morning, at the early hour of 7, they let us know that we can see a *marriage* in the Jewish quarter. Although a bit tired, I get up and dress quickly, hoping to see something like what Delacroix painted. I was not to be disappointed"[50] [**figs. 9 and 10**]. Traversing the town to reach the mellah or Jewish quarter, Charcot noted the activity of the market day, the oriental costumes everywhere, and the distinctive dress that enabled the Jewish inhabitants to be recognized "du premier coup" [**figs. 11 and 12**]. His vivid account of the wedding scene took in the interior setting and costumes, the traditional dressing of the bride by the women, the vows exchanged, the food and drink, the music and dancing. The ceremony made a powerful impression, especially the women chanting to the rhythmic beat of a tambourine that accompanied the dressing of the bride. "The overall effect is powerful and penetrating. One feels transported back centuries in time, creating the sensation of a dream."[51] This was something of a role reversal for the neurologist famous for inducing dream-like states in patients subjected to hypnosis.

Charcot's eye-witness account of the Jewish wedding invites comparison with Delacroix's description of the ceremony he witnessed in Tangiers fifty-five years earlier. While the artist immersed himself in the aesthetic features of the scene, the physician added comments informed by a medical gaze: "The eyes are beautiful in general," Charcot noted about the women, echoing the artist and the standard trope of the beautiful exotic Jewess, but then he tarnished the image: "the face is often puffy and scrofulous."[52]

What Charcot could not understand was for him "bizarre," such as the words in Hebrew or the unfamiliar meats, pastries, and beverages that he cautiously tasted. He remarked sarcastically that when it came to the ritual breaking of the wine glass, a chipped cup "more or less cleverly substitutes" for the "beautiful brand new glass."[53] Charcot's irreverent sense of humor came to the fore in his description of the bride.

> During this long torture, she remains completely motion-less—one could say she has a face of wax. Her eyes are closed. Doubtless, no expression ought to adorn the lightly made-up face on which beauty marks [*mouches*] have been placed here and there. It is painful to see the unfortunate "happy" person. What would she do if she becomes hot or if her nose starts to itch? Suffer. Would she be disowned for scratching her nose?[54]

Delacroix also noted the immobility of the bride and he too referred to her as "*malheureuse*." But the artist's sympathetic tone contrasted with clinician's detachment, illustrated by Charcot's repeated allusion to the bride as a figure of "wax" as if she had a pathological symptom similar to the "waxy immo-bility" he observed in hysterics or somnambulists.[55]

1.6 "Une race aussi originale que cette race des sémites"[56]

In general, Charcot responded negatively to the Jewish pre-sence in Tetuan. Visiting the home of a well-to-do Jewish merchant, the physician compared it unfavorably with the Moorish residences he had admired the previous day: "it is less opulent and dirtier."[57] Charcot immediately characterized his host as "an old rascal" ["*un vieux filou*"] who tried without success to soften up his visitors with refreshments hoping they would make some purchases. Adding parsimony to the stereotype of the Jew as devious and avaricious, the physician noted contemptuously that the merchant sought to obtain medical services on the cheap from his distinguished visitor. Charcot complied and examined the family. But he riposted, thinking to shame the merchant, by waiving his fees altogether. To no avail: "he couldn't care less."

More broadly, Charcot wondered why the Jews of Tetuan, who descended from the community driven out of Spain centuries earlier, continued to wear the garb and speak the language of "leurs persécuteurs."[58] On visiting the school founded by the French-based Alliance Israelite Universelle, he deplored the failure of its teachers, who had been trained in France, to preserve any sense of gratitude to the French state: "*Nothing*," he exclaimed, "they are *heimatlosen*, no homeland, at home everywhere" [emphasis in original].[59] Charcot here echoed another frequent and potent negative stereotype of the Jews as an intrinsically homeless race composed of wealthy cosmopolitans at one extreme of society and impoverished wanderers at the other.[60]

To conclude from such examples that Charcot was a confirmed anti-semite would be excessive. His prejudices regarding Jews were commonplace stereotypes, widely diffused in polite European society, not least among French intellectuals. There is no evidence to suggest that Charcot had any involvement with the organized anti-semitic movement that in the 1880s was becoming a serious force in France and elsewhere. Absent are the tropes of visceral anti-Semitism that portrayed Jews as a race of evil and rapacious exploiters of the indigenous, in this case, Arab population.[61] In referring to the separate and distinct Jewish neighborhood of Tetuan, Charcot uses a neutral generic term, "*quartier.*"

On the other hand, unlike Delacroix and many others, Charcot has nothing to say, sympathetic or otherwise, about the difficult circumstances under which Jews lived in Morocco.[62] Here, as elsewhere in the journal, the physician appears apolitical.

The Moroccan journal, however, significantly displays Charcot's keen interest in finding medical evidence supporting a pre-conceived notion of essential Jewish particularity. Ascribing traits such as *heimatlosen* to Jews as a race presumes intrinsic or natural qualities. Charcot's perception of Muslims, on the other hand, is more nuanced. In their case, he notes social class differences. On arrival at Ceuta, he sees "Moors of all kinds: peasants, bourgeoisie, merchants, black and white Moroccans."[63]

Charcot believed that his area of expertise, diseases of the nervous system and related chronic ailments, provided confirming evidence of Jewish distinctiveness.[64] In a Tuesday lesson on 23 October 1888, he declared that a young Jewish woman from the Alsace region of France, whom he had diagnosed with hysteria in a previous lesson, was an example of "the extent to which that race displays to an unmatched frequency nervous manifestations of all kinds." He went on to say,

> During a little expedition [*une petite incursion*] that I undertook in Morocco last year, I recently confirmed this fact [of Jewish pathology] once again under conditions particularly favorable to the demonstration. There, in Tetuan, nearly six thousand Jews, who were chased out of Spain three centuries ago, have lived tightly cooped up in a Ghetto. Intermarriage is the rule and thus hereditary factors accumulate, grow, and act in full force. So much so that I was able in a brief space of time to recognize within this very restricted population numerous interacting derangements belonging to the arthritic and nervous diatheses.[65]

This passage reveals that Charcot did in fact allow his pleasure trip to cross over into scientific matters and his travelogue to result in medical discourse. At Tetuan, he was able to confirm to his satisfaction certain preconceived notions about Jewish pathology. In generalizing, he neglected or ignored well-recognized differences between the Sephardic Jews whom he had observed in Morocco and the Ashkenazi Jews of Eastern Europe who constituted the majority of Jewish patients he had seen at his Salpêtrière clinic. (His reference to "ghetto" in the Tuesday lesson also suggests a conflation of Sephardim with Ashkenazim). Moreover, Charcot attributed the proliferation of various expressions of "nervous and arthritic pathology" to intermarriage and heredity.

The Moroccan journal conveys a more modest and less conclusive account of what the physician in fact observed among the Jews of Tetuan. On Thursday, August 11, Charcot examined several patients at the house of the Jewish merchant, and then, later that day, at the request of the Spanish consul and the military envoy, he consented to hold a consultation. In the first group, he noted: "These people are all eczematous, arthritic, puffy, scrofulous. Two infants a few months old have indurated and inflamed swellings in their groins. They look to me to be complications of circumcision" (A, 10-d).[66] He described his afternoon clinic as follows:

> Here come the patients, 5 or 6 of them, all Jews. They file into the patio. I sketch one who presents a beautiful case of Parkinson's [**fig. 13**]. Nothing very interesting from the point of view of diagnosis. But all are nervous cases [*des nerveux*]. Yesterday, on the square, they showed me a Jew who remained mute, so they say, during his entire childhood, but who eventually began to speak. Was he a case of hysteria? (**A, 11-a, b**)[67] [**fig. 14**]

This appears to have been the extent of Charcot's medical observations in Tetuan. Rather limited, but sufficient in his estimation to incorporate into a Tuesday lesson as persuasive support for the notion of a special Jewish pathology. Although the journal account downplayed the scientific interest of the Jewish patients, Charcot's letter to his wife written that same day was more positive: "To please the physician of the Spanish legation who has an outpatient clinic here, I gave 2 or 3 free consultations. I saw some interesting cases. What a fine thing it is to see these things up close and how instructive. I'm delighted to see that my son gets enthusiastic about all this and profits from it."[68]

Edouard Drumont, journalist and self-declared leader of the French anti-semitic movement, made use of Charcot's remarks on Jewish neurosis to legitimate his programme by invoking the leading authority on nervous diseases.[69] There is no evidence that the neurologist was involved, much less approved, of Drumont's references to him in his best-selling *La France Juive* (1886) and elsewhere. On the contrary, some perceived Charcot to be personally on good terms with Jews.[70] In 1897, in the midst of the Dreyfus Affair, Jean-Baptiste Charcot wrote to Emile Zola that his late father had detested Drumont and his "horde of anti-semites."[71]

More significant, and perhaps more revealing of Charcot's perspective, the son went on to say that his father had been preparing "for a long time a grand medico-philosophical work that he wished to entitle 'Israel.'"[72] Such an interest or "medico-philosophical" preoccupation with Jews might best be categorized as "Semitism," an ostensibly objective investigation similar to contemporary researches by Ernest Renan and many others. Rather than motivated by personal prejudice, such as Charcot displayed in his journal, or the political ideology of anti-semitism à la Drumont, such research could claim the objectivity accorded positivistic science.

Charcot's Moroccan journal situated Jews within a medical discourse that in itself was neither philo- nor anti-semitic. Similarly, his Tuesday lessons left open either possibility. "To be fair to the Jews," he declared, "drunkenness is not one of the defects of a race which, they say, has many defects, but also very great qualities."[73]

Charcot's repeated references to Jews in his *Leçons du Mardi* suggest objectives that were primarily epistemological rather than racial. From the outset of the 1880s, the neurologist increasingly claimed heredity to be the causal explanation for diseases of the nervous system and other presumably related chronic ailments.[74] To support this claim, given the undeveloped state of contemporary theories of heredity, Charcot followed his natural preference for empirical clinical investigation. He urged the collection of family genealogies of patients, dozens of which filled his *Leçons du Mardi* and subsequent publications. Among these family pedigrees of disease, the neurologist pointed to the exceptional heuristic value of the study of Jews:

> It would make a very interesting investigation to devote a special study to the diseases of a race as original as this semitic race which has played such an important role in history from antiquity to the present. That would be a very beautiful source of observations for comparative pathology.[75]

More concisely, Charcot summed up his firm belief in a research program targeting heredity in a personal letter: "well just take a look," he wrote to a skeptical (and Jewish) Sigmund Freud, "(the research is easy, *especially in Jewish families*)"[76] [emphasis in original]. He went on to say to his former pupil that he was currently directing "a campaign of this kind" demonstrating the inheritance of diabetes.[77]

Charcot's assumptions about the validity and usefulness of semitism as a medical category clearly biased his few clinical observations in Tetuan. The evidence he found there, scant as it was, struck him as "particularly favorable to the demonstration," and he incorporated the Tetuan experience into his teaching. The notion that Jews as a race had an innate predisposition toward certain diseases, especially nervous ailments, was widespread in the medical literature of the fin-de-siècle. Charcot's personal library shows that he noted with reading marks what colleagues, such as the physician, Cesare Lombroso, and the psychologist, Théodule Ribot, among others, had to say on Jews.[78] The neurologist thus should be seen as a vector for rather than an originator of vague constitutional explanations of chronic disease that began to assume a racial component in the 1880s. None of the contemporary formulations of the issue of Jewish pathology, however, carried an authority comparable to that of the leader of the Salpêtrière school, nor did they imply a comparable program of clinical investigation.[79]

1.7 A "visuel"

Charcot's Moroccan journal offers other insights in addition to what I have termed the writer's semitism. His fascination with North Africa easily qualifies as one among many specimens of European "orientalism," a celebratory idealized, even fantasized, perception of the picturesque and exotic in Eastern culture within a framework confident of Western superiority. The morning after arriving in Tetuan, despite the fatiguing journey and little sleep, Charcot felt elated and wrote to his wife, "Nevertheless, I got up around 6 in the morning, awaken by all sort of cries from the Tetuan marketplace. We are in a fantasy world here, a real tale from the thousand and one nights come to life. Nothing jarring, everything exotic and pure."[80] On an earlier excursion into the mountains, on first crossing into Morocco, he exclaimed, "Africa, true Africa. Like yesterday [seeing] the cork oak trees, the black palms, the oleanders when there is a river, etc. etc.—in short, the real thing."[81]

Charcot's quest for "l'Afrique vraie" where each element of nature corresponded to its ideal type is reminiscent of his search as a clinician for pure types of neurological ailments, waiting for the researcher to discover by careful observation. The Moroccan journal is replete with instances of this mode of observation in which Charcot discerns a prototype underlying, for example, various architectural forms (mosques, residences, patterns of tiles, and mosaics) and his dismay when encountering a false note. His identification of Tetuan with Granada, "Farewell, daughter of Granada; we shall soon pay a pious visit to your mother . . . Tetuan is Granada and Granada is Tetuan" **(A, 14-b, 15-d)**,[82] shows the same attention to ideal types that was characteristic of his clinical project to create order from a chaos of clinical observations and to construct nosography from structural details ultimately founded on hereditary transmission.[83]

The journal provides a rare, if not unique, first-person account of Charcot's inner thoughts. As Sigmund Freud remarked, his mentor was not a profound thinker but rather a "*visuel,*" a "see-er" (in the double meaning of one who sees and a visionary who sees beyond appearances) who relied primarily on observation and a remarkable ability to think by means of visualization.[84] In addition to this common sense meaning of *visuel,* Freud referred to a technical category of language acquisition that Charcot himself had been one of the first to describe. In his work on various types of aphasias or language disorders, Charcot had defined corresponding psychological types of which the *visuel* was one of three innate possibilities.[85]

Freud's remark finds ample confirmation in Charcot's record of his Moroccan voyage. Here one finds the "searching gaze" ["*œil scrutateur*"] (8-c) hard at work, even though the neurologist is, for the most part, on vacation.[86] Significantly, the verb "to see" ["*voir*"] is employed nearly forty times in the absence of a first person voice (*on voit, se voit, il faut voir, laisse voir,* etc.) as compared with only five times in the active form (*je vois*) thus underscoring the putative objectivity of the observer who transmits what is seen or to be seen.

Charcot explicitly invokes the painter's eye by using the word "painting" ["*tableau*"] twice and again by his desire to see a scene which Delacroix painted. More often he implies the visual mode with vivid descriptions of landscapes analyzed like pictures[87] and by frequent use of words such as "*l'effet*" ("the mass of white tombstones creates an effect of white laundry drying in the open air"[88] and "*l'air*" ("who looks like a big fool," "looks to be a sacristan of the synagogue"[89] (A, 4-b, 4-c) [emphasis added].[90] By comparison, the other senses are seldom evoked.[91] Even in one of his several descriptions of toilet facilities, Charcot puts the sense of sight before smell: "It is perfect, a paradise for the senses of sight and smell"[92] (A, 8-d).

The Moroccan journal as a whole conveys a passion to see. This, rather than any particular conceptual or literary merits, makes it a remarkable record. Except for this quality and the historical importance of a figure whose personality remains somewhat enigmatic, the journal would otherwise simply be one among several accounts by nineteenth-century French tourists who ventured to go beyond Tangiers in Morocco.

Charcot's journal is a series of finely drawn word pictures, the verbal counterpart of sketches and the recreational analogue of the neurologist's working method. When he declares, after his consultation with patients, that he wants to see the panorama of Tetuan one last time so as to carry away "an indelible visual impression,"[93] Charcot tacitly acknowledges the priority of the visual over the written record. And, in the journal's final sentence, he comments on the ease with which a little imagination ["*un petit effort de vision interne*"] (**A, 15-d**) could transform present-day Tetuan into the Granada of four centuries ago.

The culmination of the visit to Tetuan comes with Charcot on the terrace of the fonda Espagnole on the morning of departure, sketching a view of the town as he seeks to inscribe his images of the previous days: "All that returns to mind as I do my sketch . . . I would relish doing another sketch for I am in fine form [*en verve*]" (**A, 13-d**)[94] [**fig. 16**]. Earlier in the voyage, he had written to his wife that despite his feeling "that old age is beginning to blunt the liveliness of new impressions for me, I have to say that I have been moved profoundly by everything . . ."[95] If, for Charcot, seeing was the pathway to thinking, the journal of his Moroccan voyage provides a rich record of his distinctive mode of perception.

NOTES

1. Sigmund Freud, "Charcot," in *The Standard Edition of the Complete Psychological Works*, trans. and ed. by James Strachey, vol. 3, 11–23. Freud began his eulogy of his former teacher: "The young science of neurology has lost its greatest leader, neurologists of every country have lost their master teacher and France has lost one of her foremost men." Freud's eulogy was dated August 1893, the month of Charcot's death.
2. Ibid., 11.
3. See Christopher G. Goetz, Michel Bonduelle, and Toby Gelfand, *Charcot: Constructing Neurology*, (New York: Oxford University Press, 1995).

4. "Ce bon vieil hospice de la Salpêtrière." Charcot in "Banquet offert à M. le professeur Charcot," *Le Progrès Médical*, 8 décembre 1883, 1000.

5. Octave Mirbeau, "Le siècle de Charcot" in *Chroniques du diable*, ed. Pierre Michel (*Annales littéraires de l'Université de Besançon*, 555, Diffusion les Belles Lettres: Paris, 1995), 121–27. Mirbeau's article first appeared anonymously in *L'Événément* (29 May 1885).

6. See note 38 below for Charcot's pleasure at being recognized by the general public.

7. Letter of Kinnosuke Miura to Charcot (1893), Bibliothèque Charcot, Archives, MAVIII 6, chemise 7.

8. See Goetz, Bonduelle, and Gelfand, 218–22, 296–300, 311–12; and Bonduelle, "Charcot et l'Italie," *Neurologia Psichiatria Scienze Umane* 17 (1997): 179–89.

9. Charcot's zest for England, despite the seriousness of this mission, was irrepressible. On the eve of his departure in June 1893, he wrote to Sigmund Freud: "I leave immediately for London where I will refortify myself a bit with Shakespeare." See Gelfand, "'Mon cher docteur Freud': Charcot's unpublished correspondence to Freud, 1888–1893." *Bulletin of the History of Medicine* 62 (1988): 575.

10. A fireworks display at the London Congress honored Charcot by projecting his image into the sky along with those of two colleagues representing Great Britain and Germany as he did France. He exulted privately to his wife: "J'ai ici un véritable triomphe que je partage avec Mr Pasteur. Lui et moi nous représentons le groupe Français." Letter August 8, 1881. Vallin-Charcot family archives. Housed at Neuilly-sur-Seine, consisting of personal correspondance and other documents (uncatalogued). Hereafter cited as Charcot family papers.

11. Sergines, "Les échos de Paris," *Les Annales politiques et littéraires* 21 (27 août, 1893): 133. According to the author of this brief but well-informed obituary notice, Charcot used to say when called on a consultation outside of Paris: "Je suis content! je vais à X . . . Je pourrai du même coup, soulager une souffrance et . . . visiter le musée de X . . . qui, dit-on est fort beau!"; Charcot published with his student, Paul Richer, *Les démoniaques dans l'art*, (Paris:

Delahaye et Lecrosnier, 1887), and *Les difformes et les malades dans l'art*, (Paris: Lecrosnier et Babé, 1889).

12. Charcot traveled to Madrid and Malaga with another Paris professor on a consultation at the end of December 1887. In 1888, he spent periods in Northern Italy and elsewhere as medical advisor to the ailing Emperor of Brazil, Don Pedro. See Charcot family papers.

13. In 1880, in the course of a month-long visit to Spain, Charcot had considered but then abandoned the project of crossing to Tangiers. In January 1889, he traveled to Algiers to aid his ailing brother, and found time to visit the city as well. Charcot family papers. According to one of his students, Henry Meige, Charcot visited other sites in North Africa, including Sousse and Tripoli, but the family archives do not corroborate Meige's testimony. *Étude sur certains Névropathes Voyageurs. Le Juif errant à la Salpêtrière*, (Paris, thesis, 1893).

14. The travel journal in the Charcot family papers consists of two separate portions. The longer, which I have designated "A," contains fifteen numbered manuscript sheets each folded into four pages, here identified for reference as a, b, c, d. The obvious gap in the narrative in manuscript "A" between sheets 2 and 3 is filled by manuscript "B" consisting of nine sheets bearing the numbers 3 to 11. Again each sheet is folded into four pages. The pages are 18 cm by 11 cm. "B" is preceded by a page bearing the title, *huit jours au Maroc. Ceuta et Tetuan*. Charcot wrote the journal on his personal stationery. The first two sheets of "A" bear a printed "17, Quai Malaquais," his former Paris address, while the remainder have "217, Boulevard St-Germain," his current address to which he moved in 1884. "B" is written entirely on "217, Boulevard St-Germain" stationary except for the title page.

15. *Leçons du mardi à la Salpêtrière: Policlinique 1887–88, 1888–89*, 2 vols. (Paris: Progrès Médical, 1887, 1889, 1892). See Gelfand, "Mon cher docteur Freud": 563–88.

16. See below Moroccan journal (**A, 6-b**). See also Charcot's encounter with "les dames" (**B, 4-a, b**), and his reunion with Burty at the end of the voyage (**A, 15-b, c**). His remark about camels in

the marketplace, "ça tient de la place un chameau" ["A camel takes up space, it does"] (**A, 6-a**), sounded a droll note worthy of a dead-pan comedian. A contemporary noted this lighter side of "le maître": "Charcot, quoique généralement silencieux, avait de violents accès de gaieté. Sa gaieté, un peu bourrue, éclatait alors en boutades, fort piquantes . . . " *Les Annales politiques et littéraires* 21 (1893, 27 août): 133. Henry Meige, "Charcot Artiste," *Nouvelle Iconographie de la Salpêtrière* 11 (1898): 508, also noted that Charcot revealed to his intimates a Rabelaisian sense of humor: "il aimait la grosse farce. Il citait volontiers de mémoire des passages de Rabelais."

17. The family's correspondence from Morocco is in the Bibliothèque Charcot, Charcot Archives, MA VIII 2 pacquet 3 "Voyage en Afrique – 1887."

18. Eugene Delacroix, *Souvenirs d'un voyage dans le Maroc*, édition de Laure Beaumont-Maillet, Barthélémy Jobert et Sophie Join-Lambert, (Paris: Gallimard, 1999).

19. See Meige, "Charcot Artiste," 489–516.

20. Charcot family papers. Delacroix gave instructions in his will for Burty to prepare a catalogue for the sale of his drawings. He published this in 1864 and an edition of Delacroix's letters in 1878. On Philippe Burty (1830–1890), see G. Vapereau, *Dictionnaire des contemporains*, 5 ed., (Paris: 1880), 334. See also Burty, "Eugène Delacroix au Maroc," *Gazette des Beaux-Arts* 19 (1865), and H. Bessis, "Philippe Burty et Eugène Delacroix," *Gazette des Beaux-Arts* (1968): 195–202. In his own will, Burty left Charcot his Delacroix album of the voyage to Morocco along with several photographs of Delacroix's watercolors. See *Journal de Eugène Delacroix*, ed. Paul Flat et René Piot, t. 1 (1823–1850), (Paris: Plon, 1893, 145 n. 2). This first publication of Delacroix's journal and subsequent editions did not reproduce the drawings in the original that Charcot would have seen. A complete facsimile of the carnets de voyage de Maroc was published only in 1992. Among other preparations for Morocco, Charcot evidently consulted newspaper and other contemporary accounts. For Tetuan, he mentions the article in the Larousse encyclopedic

dictionary, Vapereau's dictionary, and he noted: "Tetuan -cité dans Don Quichotte."

21. "Espérant voir quelque chose comme ce qu'a peint Delacroix. Je ne devais pas être trompé" (**Ms A 3-a**).

22. *Leçons du mardi*, vol. 2, 12.

23. "*nous nous fouillons partout où nous avons accès d'un œil scrutateur*" (**Ms A, 8-c**).

24. "*Rien ne dépare le tableau si ce n'est nous et nous ne nous regardons pas. . . . Notre passage n'a produit aucune émotion, nulle part*" (**A, 3-a, 3-b**).

25. "*Nous ne sommes pas ici pour nous amuser – bravez toutes les vermines de la création: cela fait partie du programme*" (**A, 2-b**).

26. "*Prêts à faire quelque mauvais coup*" (**A, 14-c**). In a letter to his mother, Jean-Baptiste Charcot mentioned his father's high spirits on their sea voyage: "le patron enveloppé dans un caoutchau à Buison n'a pas reçu un goutte d'eau et a blagué tout le temps" (Letter August 13, Algeciras).

27. "*Par notre inépuisable appétit . . . on n'aura jamais vu faire tant des repas et de repas si copieux! Décidemment cette cure d'exercice corporel au grand air, par une température moyenne de 35 à l'ombre est chose à conseiller*" (**A, 11-c**).

28. To his wife, he wrote that the music was "*atroce*" (Letter of August 13). Although Charcot had an extensive familiarity with Western classical music, he evidently shared the disdain of the Arabic music expressed by French travelers to the Middle East. See Jean-Claude Berchet, Introduction, *Le voyage en Orient*, (Robert Laffont: 1985).

29. Nothing in Charcot's published works supports a deeper interpretation of Freud's often-cited phrase attributed to his teacher: "c'est toujours la chose génitale, toujours . . . toujours . . . toujours," Freud, *On the History of the Psycho-analytic Movement* (1914) in *The Standard Edition of the Complete Psychological Works*, trans. and ed. by James Strachey, vol. 14, 14; Charcot insisted on his own "impeccability" in sexual matters, in contrast to the behavior of a traveling companion. In a letter of 19 February 1889 written from Algiers to his wife, he stated: "Ce soir j'ai parcouru la ville arabe. Je me croyais à Tetuan. Seulement ici on entre partout, et même

nous avons pénètre dans quelques intérieurs fort équivoques où Legendre a couru de grands dangers; mais sa vertu je dois le dire n'a pas succombé. J'ajoutai que c'était tellement dégoûtant qu'il n'y a pas eu grand mérite. Je ne parle pas de moi, bien entendu . . . je suis absolument impeccable" (Charcot family papers).

30. Charcot family papers. On this Spanish phase of the voyage, Charcot gives an account in his album of his "Visite à l'Hôpital provincial de S. Lazaro para los enfermos de Elephantias" at Seville and the conditions ("veritablement affreux . . . ignobles") of thirty lepers in a ward at the Hôpital Général in Granada.

31. Arène, a friend and frequent traveling companion of Charcot and his children, is only mentioned once in the journal as the group bids farewell to Burty and him. But a letter from Charcot to his wife makes clear that Arène in fact incited Burty to desert: "Nous avons laissé à Algesiras le lâche Burty. Une conversation qu'il avait eu la veille avec l'hypochondriaque Arène sur le vent d'est, sur les difficultés de la traverse dans le détroit, sur le mal de mer enfin l'ont complètement retourné et il a demandé grâce. Grâce que je lui ai accordé: mais voilà – un brave homme condamné à tout jamais comme voyageur" (Lettre de Ceuta, 8 aout 1887). Charcot's reference to a "consul hypochondriaque" (**A, 15-b**) suggests that the "Arène" here was not Paul but his brother Jules, who was in the French diplomatic service in North Africa. In any case, Charcot in his letter reveals a stronger tone of dominating the travel party than in the journal where he merely agrees not to "insister" against Burty's decision to remain behind.

32. Letter to Mme Charcot, 13 August 1887, Algesiras. I follow Charcot's orthography in the spelling of "Tetuan," which was usually written in French as "Tétouan" and similarly in English. See note 33 for the quotation.

33. Letter from Wednesday [August 10] appended to a letter by Jeanne Charcot to Mme Charcot: "Tetuan est une perle, un bijou – c'est complet! Tanger est m'assure t-on une ville sans caractère. Il y a 20,000 espagnols; à Tetuan il n'y en a pas 20. Donc nous brûlons Tanger, pour gagner du temps." The historian, Jean-Louis Miège, *Le Maroc et l'Europe (1830–1894)*, (Paris:

Presses Universitaires de France, 1963), t. 4,286, n. 1, notes that there were about 3,000 Spanish in Tangier and about 200 in Tetuan, according to the consular census in 1887, the same year as Charcot's trip. Although Charcot's estimates were thus grossly inaccurate, his qualitative contrast is confirmed. Charcot probably took his other estimates of the population groups in Tetuan from his reading of the Larousse entry on the town. For other contemporary descriptions of Tetuan and Morocco see H.P. de LaMartinière, *La Grande Encyclopédie*, t. 23 [1896]: 242–79, and "Lettres de Maroc," *Le Temps*, written at monthly intervals by the newspaper's correspondent in Tangier. The article "Tetuan" *Encyclopedia Britannica*, 11 ed. (1910), vol. 26, 672 by Kate A. Meakin is also informative. France had a consul general in Tangiers and an agent consulaire in Tetuan, but the Charcot party relied upon and fraternized with the Spanish authorities. Jean-Baptiste wrote to his mother: "Le séjour à Tetuan en plein Maroc sans plus de huit Européens tous d'un très-grande amabilité d'ailleurs a été délicieux" (Letter of 13 August 1887).

34. *"une vraie ville arabe telle qu'on ne la verait pas en Algérie ou à Tunis. C'est neuf, tous neuf."* Charcot letter, 13 August 1887.

35. Maurice Paléologue, "Le Maroc. Notes et Souvenirs," *Revue des Deux Mondes* 83 (15 avril, 1885): 888–924, esp. 888–889. Paléologue's voyage took place over three months in the beginning of 1883. Another commentator of the same period observed: "L'Algérie, la Tunisie, l'Egypte, sont des pays ouverts aux touristes, et on s'y promène pour son agrément. Longtemps encore, l'empire du Maroc n'attirera que les voyageurs sérieux, qui ont toutes les petites et les grandes vertues de leur profession." G. Valbert, "Un Voyageur Français au Maroc," *Revue des Deux Mondes* 86 (1 avril, 1888): 670–81, esp. 670. According to Miège, 295, n. 1, tourism to Morocco could only be said to have begun *after 1887* with the installation of multiple steam ship lines. The first two tourist guidebooks appeared the following year.

36. See Barthélémy Jobert, *Delacroix*, (Paris: Gallimard, 1997), 139–76.

37. "Voilà la disposition du terrain de Ceuta à Tctuan. Pas de route proprement dit d'ailleurs. Des sentiers à peine tracés ; pas

d'arbres, des buissons plus ou moins touffus et plus ou moins élevés représentants parfois de petits bois en miniature . . . Pas de villages c'est le désert" (**B, 6-d**). The writer, Pierre Loti, traveling from Tangiers to Tetuan less than two years after Charcot, described the terrain in nearly the same terms: "Pas de routes au Maroc, jamais, nulle part; des espèces de sentiers de chèvres, avec le droit de passer à gué les rivières qui se présentent . . . pas une route, pas un village, pas une maison, pas un campement; la terre restée dans sa splendeur première." *Cette éternelle nostalgie. Journal intime (1878–1911)*, édition établie, présentée et annotée par Bruno Vercier, Alain Quella-Villeger et Guy Dugas, (Paris: La Table Ronde, 1997), 261–62. Loti was invited to accompany the mission of the new minister of France at Tangiers to the sultan of Maroc at Fez in the spring of 1889.

38. "On me présente comme un personnage" (**B 4-b**). Charcot took obvious pride in being recognized even by the humble in Tetuan: "on rencontre un cordonnier arabe qui dit à Jean qu'il me connaissait par une photographie et qu'il m'a vu passer dans la rue" (Letter to Mme Charcot, 13 August 1887).

39. "Nous voilà loin d'Europe, de France, de Paris . . . ici rien de banal . . . lieux presqu'inexplorés . . . Hélas un fragment de journal jauni git à terre . . . J'y lis en gros caractère, Le Figaro !!!" (**A, 8-d**).

40. "Quelques unes de ces grosses boules brillantes argentées dont les bourgeois sans goût de notre pays ornent nos jardins" (**A, 7-b-c**).

41. Charcot remarked about a wealthy Moorish home that the group visited: "ici la collection de glaces et de pendules est des plus riches; c'est affreux. Mais nous collectionons les bibelots des autres; pourquoi ne collectionnerait-t-on pas les nôtres" (**A, 9-c**).

42. Goncourt, *Journal. Mémoires de la vie littéraire*, (Paris: Robert Lafont: 1989), vol. 2, 823 (1879, 26 mai). For an insightful and fairer discussion of the Charcot family's artistic taste and their considerable personal artisanal skills, see Deborah Silverman, *Art Nouveau in Fin-de-Siècle France*, (Berkeley: University of California Press, 1989), esp. 75–108. Their workmanship can still be seen at their summer country home at Neuilly-sur-Seine,

which remains the residence of Charcot's great granddaughter, and has been classed as an historic site.

43. "Je m'installe comme un infirme que je suis . . . Jeanne a les infirmités naturelles à son sexe" (**B, 4-b, 6-b**).

44. Jeanne Charcot described the caravan that departed Ceuta at 5:30 AM: "Nous sommes partis sur cinq mulets trois autres mulets portaient les sacs les tentes et les provisions, deux Maures appartenant à l'armée espagnole en grand costume, deux autres Arabes du Maroc armés, et un nègre du plus beau noir formaient notre escorte, de plus trois muletiers."

45. "On commence à tancer les maures de l'empereur qui nous ont conduit par ce mauvais chemin" (**B, 7-c**). Charcot wrote to assure his wife before their departure: "Mais ce n'est que demain que doit avoir lieu la fameuse expédition à Tétouan. C'est difficile, mais cela me parait faisable. Je vois aucun danger surtout" (Letter from Ceuta, 8 August 1887).

46. "Chiens de chrétiens, il est trop tard . . . allez vous coucher . . . en plein air" (**B, 10-b-c**).

47. "Grand, maigre très prévenant, orné d'une cravate impossible et d'un gilet blanc interminable qui mettent bien en relief sa bonne figure de Don Quichotte."

48. "Ces pauvres bêtes" (**A, 2-d**).

49. "Papa m'étonne, il embarque, il débarque d'un canot dans un autre il monte et il descend de mulet, il y reste 13 heures et il peut encore sortir à 6 h. 1/2 du matin!" Letter, Wednesday [August 10].

50. "Le lendemain matin de bonne heure 7 heures on vient nous dire qu'il y a à voir une *noce* dans le quartier juif. Quoique un peu fatigué je me lève et m'habille rapidement espérant voir quelque chose comme ce qu'a peint Delacroix. Je ne devais pas être trompé" (**A, 3-a**) [emphasis in original].

51. "Tout cela est pénétrant, on se sent transporter plusieurs siècles en arrière – ça fait l'effet d'un rêve" (**A, 4-a**). Paléologue described the mental effects of music he heard in the mellah at Marakesh: "produisait d'abord sur l'oreille un effet d'agacement et de lassitude, mais s'imposait peu à peu à l'esprit et

s'en emparait impérieusement . . . Comme sous l'influence du hachich, mais avec une moindre intensité, le cerveau se sent lentement pris par ces ondulations sonores, toujours les mêmes, qui viennent le frapper dans le même rythme et dans le même ordre. Au bout d'une demi-heure de cette musique étrange, on se sent en un état d'esprit qui fait comprendre les longues extases des derviches; on trouve un charme enivrant au chant que perçoit l'oreille, et toutes sortes d'images oubliées et de rêves lointains apparaissent à travers la fumée des brûle-parfums" (Paléologue, 913).

52. "Les yeux sont beaux en général, la face souvent bouffie et strumeuse" (A, 3-b). Delacroix's initial impression of the Jewish women was that they were "perles d'Eden" (Lettre à Pierret, 25 janvier 1832, in *Correspondance*, ed. Burty, Paris 1880, vol. 1, 174). The Larousse article "Tetuan, " t. 15 (Paris, 1876): "les filles d'Israel, aussi bien celles de Tétouan que celles de Tanger n'ont pas de rivales en beauté; leurs yeux et leurs pieds sont admirables . . ." Charles Didier, an early French visitor to Tetuan, wrote "les femmes juives ont échappe à la dégénération dont les hommes sont frappes; elles sont aussi belles qu'ils sont laids . . . Toutes les Juives ont de beaux yeux noirs pleins de flamme, et la peau très blanche" (*Revue des Deux Mondes*, 8 novembre 1836, 260).

53. "Plus ou moins habilement" for the "beau verre tout neuf" (A, 4-c).

54. "Pendant ce long supplice elle garde une immobilité systématique – on dirait une figure de cire. Les yeux sont fermé. Aucune expression sans doute ne doit se peindre sur la figure légèrement fardée et sur laquelle on a placé ça et là des mouches. La malheureuse ou bienheureuse fait peine à voir. Doit elle avoir chaud et si une démangeaison lui venait au nez . . . que faire? Souffrir. Serait-elle répudiée pour avoir gratté son nez? " (A, 4a -b).

55. Delacroix described the bride: "Rien n'est singulier comme la marche de cette malheureuse qui, les paupières toujours closes, semble ne faire aucun mouvement qui naisse de sa propre volonté. Ses traits sont aussi impossibles devant cette procession que pendant tout le temps de ses autres épreuves. On m'a assuré que pour

la faire manquer à ce sérieux imperturbable, on pousse la malice jusqu'à la pincer en route. Je crois que c'est très rare qu'on voie ces pauvres créatures donner le moindre signe d'impatience ou seulement d'attention à tout ce qui se passe" (Delacroix, "Une Noce Juive dans le Maroc," *Magasin Pittoresque* 10 (1842): 30). Strictly speaking, both Delacroix and Charcot witnessed the preparations of the wedding rather than the entire ceremony. Charcot wrote to his wife: "J'ai eu ce matin la chance d'assister aux préparatif d'un mariage juif, dans le ghetto. Je te raconterai cela en détails: cela en vaut la peine. Costumes cérémonies, chantes bizarres. Nous avons du prendre part à un repas où nous avons gouté au bout des lèvres force mets bizarres et des boissons étranges – chants des siècles passés *etc etc* Être aussi transporté dans un monde étrange et original, vaut bien la peine que nous nous sommes donnés" (Lettre de mercredi [10 aout]). Another French artist, Alfred Dehodencq, painted sympathetically a number of scenes of Jewish life in Tetuan in the 1850s, including a wedding. See Gaston Séailles, *A Dehodencq*, 2 ed., (Paris: Société de Propagation des livres d'art, 1910), esp. 124–27.

56. Charcot, *Leçons du mardi*, vol. 1, 6 (15 novembre 1887).

57. "C'est moins luxueux et c'est plus sale" (**A, 10-c**).

58. "Les Juifs de Tetuan étaient en effet les juifs venant de Castille d'ou ils ont été chassés" (**A, 3-3**). The reference is to the Sephardic Jewish community exiled from Spain in 1492.

59. "Ce sont des *heimatlosen* – pas de patrie. La patrie partout" (**A, 10-d**). Charcot employs the German *heimatlosen* to convey a stronger sense of inherent homelessness than rendered by any French (or English) equivalent.

60. At the same time, and in apparent contradiction, Charcot, as we have seen, took the Tetuan Jews to task for their persistant loyalty to a Hapsburg Empire that had sent them into exile centuries earlier.

61. See Guy de Maupassant's repellant description of the Jewish merchants he encountered in the interior of Algeria in 1881. "Ré Zar'ez," 1884. Maupassant contrasted these rapacious "hideous" Jews with "our friends and neighbors," their Europeans

counterparts. Retrieved *from Maupassant Œuvres sous TACTweb.*
(8 August 2010, <http://www.etudes-francaises.net/nefbase/
maupassant.htm>). One of the earliest French visitors to Morocco,
Charles Didier, used the whole panoply of negative stereotypes
in his account of the mellah of Tetuan. Except for their beautiful daughters, Didier considered the Jews ugly physically and
morally, filthy, servile, selfish, cowardly, mercenary, a homeless
people constituting a disloyal state within the state, holding a
secret hatred for Christians and killers of Christ (*Revue des Deux
Mondes* 8 (1836 novembre): 257–69, esp. 267).

62. Charcot used the word "*distingué*" four times in his journal to
describe the physical presence of Moroccans. In each case – the
son of a chief (**B, 5-b**), the old Moor (**B, 7-c**), merchants (**A, 7-a**),
a wealthy Moor (**A, 12-c**) – he referred to Muslims. Delacroix,
Souvenirs, 106, 112–14, 137, displayed remarkable sensitivity to the
situation of the Jews; see also Paléologue, 911–13. Nonetheless,
Paléologue remarked of his visit to the mellah at Marakesh: "toute
cette misère qui, – je ne sais pourquoi, – parait plus repoussante
sur des types juifs que sur des types de race arabe . . ." Even
Didier's strongly anti-Jewish account described the extensive legal
and social discrimination they had to endure. For an unambi-
guous example of literary anti-semitism targeted against North
African Jews, see Alphonse Daudet, "A Milianah" (1864) in *Lettres
de mon Moulin,* (Paris: Le Livre de Poche, 1991), 168–81. Daudet
based this short story upon his visit to Algeria in 1861–62.

63. "Des maures de toute condition: paysans, bourgeois, marchands:
des marocains noirs et blancs" (**A, 2-a**). Charcot, like other
European visitors, had lesser accessibility to Muslims than to
Jews. Muslims did not avail themselves of local physicians' free
medical services, nor did they come to Charcot's public consultation in Tetuan. They did not attend the school Charcot visited.
His journal has sketches only of Jews. Artists, such as Delacroix,
had difficulty obtaining Muslim women as models, a reason
for his numerous depictions of Jewish women in Tangiers. See
Correspondance de Henri Regnault, ed. Arthur Duparc, 2 ed., (Paris:
Charpentier, 1873), 346–47.

64. Similarly, Charcot and his students would reduce the medieval legend of the "wandering Jew" as well as the socio-historical reality of Jewish vagrancy to a neurosis. See below, note 79.

65. *Leçons du Mardi*, vol. 2, 11–12. "J'ai récemment constaté le fait une fois de plus, dans des conditions particulièrement favorables à la démonstration, lors d'une petite incursion que j'ai faite, l'an passé au Maroc. Là, à Tétouan, près de six mille Juifs, chassés d'Espagne il y a trois siècles, vivent depuis lors, strictement claquemurés dans un Ghetto. Les mariages consanguins y sont la règle et, par conséquent, les influences héréditaires accumulées, s'y développent et agissent dans toute leur énergie. Si bien que, dans un court espace de temps, il m'a été permis, sur une population en somme très restreinte, de reconnaître maintes fois les nombreux méfaits des diathèses arthritique et nerveuse entrant en combinaison."

66. "Tous ces gens là sont eczemateux arthritiques, bouffis, strumeux – 2 enfants de quelques mois ont dans l'aine des ganglions indurés et enflammés. Cela me parait être des accidents de la circoncision."

67. "Voilà les malades qui arrivent. Il est venu 5 ou 6, tous juifs. Ils s'accummulent dans le patio. J'en croque un qui offre un bel exemple de Parkinson. – rien de bien intéressant au point de vue de la nosographie ; mais tous sont des nerveux – hier sur la place on m'a montré un juif qui était resté muet dit on pendant toute son enfance et qui a fini par parler. Était-ce un hystérique ?"

68. "J'ai donné ici 2 ou 3 consultations gratuites à des Juifs, pour faire plaisir au médecin de la légation espagnole qui a ici un dispensaire – J'ai vu des cas curieux – quelle belle chose que de voir les choses de près et comme cela instruit. Je vois avec grand plaisir que mon fils mord à tout cela et qu'il s'en profite." Letter to Mme Charcot added to Jeanne's letter [**fig. 14**]. Twenty-year old Jean-Baptiste Charcot was at the outset of his medical studies, for which he displayed decidedly less enthusiasm than his father wished. Jean-Baptiste referred briefly to this medical experience in Tetuan in a letter to mother: "N[ou]s venons d'assister à quelques consultations donnés par le patron a de bons petits juifs dont, je crois, il t'envoie un exemplaire" (Letter J.-B. Charcot [n.d.]).

69. Drumont, *La France Juive* (Paris: Marpon and Flammarion, 1886), vol. 1, 106 and *La fin d'un monde* (Paris: Savine, 1889), xvii. See Jan Goldstein, "The Wandering Jew and the Problem of Psychiatric Anti-semitism in Fin-de-Siècle France" in *Journal of Contemporary History*, 20 (1985): 521–52 and Gelfand, "From Religious to Bio-Medical Anti-Semitism: The Career of Jules Soury" in *French Medical Culture in the Nineteenth Century*, ed. A. La Berge and M. Feingold, (Amsterdam and Atlanta, 1994), 248–79, esp. 259–61.

70. See Léon Daudet, *Panorama de la IIIe Republique*, (Paris: Gallimard, 1936), 88. Charcot had cordial social and professional relations with many French and European Jews.

71. "Combien de fois n'ai je point entendre mon père ... fulminer contre la horde anti-française des anti-sémites!" (Letter of J-B Charcot to Zola, 1 December 1897, in Zola papers, Bibliothèque nationale de France, NAF 24517, fols. 82–83). Goldstein, "The Wandering Jew," has suggested that Jean-Baptiste Charcot betrayed a sense of embarrassment and guilt over the father's association with the Jewish question and a wish, in any case, to distance the neurologist from Drumont and anti-semitism. But I think Goldstein's conclusion: "the anti-semitic accents of Charcot's psychiatric pronouncements are unmistakable" (546) is problematic. As an anticlerical Republican, the senior Charcot had reason to reject Drumont's campaign on both counts, as well as for its virulent anti-semitism.

72. "Depuis longtemps un grand ouvrage médico-philosophique qu'il voulait intituler 'Israél'" (J.-B. Charcot letter to Zola). No trace of this work can be found. Charcot's library indicates that he read attentively various general studies on Jews, such as Théodore Reinach, *Histoire des Israélites* (Paris: Hachette, 1885).

73. "C'est une justice a rendre aux juifs que l'ivrognerie n'est pas un défaut de la race, qui a dit-on bien des défauts, mais qui a aussi de bien grandes qualités" (*Leçons du mardi*, 7 février 1888, vol. 1, 196). The wording here – "dit-on" for "défauts" as opposed to the simple declarative for "grandes qualités" – might be interpreted as Charcot distancing himself from the first and

associating himself with the second position. This Tuesday lesson appears only in the first edition of the *Leçons du Mardi*.

74. See Gelfand, "Charcot's response to Freud's rebellion," *Journal of the History of Ideas* 50 (1989): 293–307.

75. "Les Sémites ont en effet ce privilège de présenter à un degré extrêmement accentué tout ce qui peut se voir en matière d'arthritisme, tout ce qu'on peut imaginer en fait d'affection neuropathique, et ce serait un travail fort intéressant à faire que d'étudier spécialement les maladies d'une race aussi originale que cette race des sémites qui a joue un si grand rôle dans le monde depuis l'antiquité jusqu' à nos jours. Il y aurait là une très belle source d'observation de pathologie comparée" (*Leçons du mardi*, vol. 1, 6, 15 November 1887). Charcot called for this study of Jews in the first lesson of the first published volume of Tuesday Lessons and repeated it frequently. See ibid, vol. 1, 110 (17 janvier 1888); 408 (10 juillet 1888); vol. 2, 11 (23 octobre 1888). Drumont quoted this initial statement in full in *Le fin d'un Monde*, xvii.

76. "Eh bien regardez y (*surtout dans les familles juives l'exploration est facile*)" (Letter, Charcot to Freud, 30 June 1892, Freud Archives, Washington D.C., in Gelfand, "Mon cher docteur Freud," 574).

77. Ibid. In 1891–92 two of Charcot's assistants published an article in his *Archives de Neurologie* that included thirty-eight family trees of diabetics. Nearly one-third bore the label "famille israélite." Georges Guinon and A. Souques, "Association du tabès avec le diabète sucré," *Archives de neurologie* (1891) and (1892): reprinted in Charcot, *Clinique des maladies du système nerveux*, ed. G. Guinon, (Paris: Progrès Médical, 1893), vol. 2, 289–348. Guinon and Souques remarked that Charcot conducted systematic genealogical research "on nearly all of the patients" who came to the out-patient clinic (ibid., 345). During his final year of teaching, Charcot returned to the subject. According to an eye-witness account, he noted that the persecutions Jews had endured over the centuries might have predisposed them to nervous diseases. Jane B. Henderson, "Personal reminiscences of M. Charcot," *Glasgow Medical Journal* 40 (1893): 293–98. Charcot had previously

invoked this notion of inherited trauma in a Tuesday lesson when he presented a patient whom he called a "wandering Jew." Racial inheritance, an aspect of the widely held Lamarckian theory of heredity, along with consanguineous marriage, formed the slender theoretical framework with which Charcot and others sought to explain Jewish pathology.

78. Bibliothèque Charcot, La Salpêtrière. Charcot's copy of the French translation of Lombroso, *L'Homme de Génie*, (Paris, 1889) bears extensive reader's marks on the discussion of Jews, 175–79 and a handwritten "Juif" in the margin, 175. Similarly, Charcot placed a handwritten marker, "Juif," at the discussion of diabetes and Jews on his copy of Charles Bouchard, *Maladies par ralentissement de la nutrition*, (Paris: Savy, 1882),185. Charcot's copy of Ribot, *L'Hérédité Psychologique*, 2ᵉ ed. (Paris: Bailliere, 1882) also bears reading marks on the discussion of Jews and mental illness (127).

79. The fullest published expression of the Salpêtrière school's views on Jewish pathology was an inaugural medical thesis supervised by Charcot [**fig. 15**]. Henry Meige, *Étude sur certains Névropathes Voyageurs. Le Juif errant à la Salpêtrière* (Paris, 1893), referred to his mentor's vast experience on the subject "basée sur des centaines de faits," presumably Jewish patients whom Charcot had treated. Yet Meige produced just five case histories, all of Russian or Eastern European origins (Meige, *Etude*, 7). He began with the one who had inspired the thesis, "Klein," a young Hungarian whom Charcot had presented to a Tuesday lesson on 19 February 1889 as "un véritable descendant d'Ahasverus ou Cartaphilus," the wandering Jew of Christian legend, now revealed by Charcot to be a case of traumatic hysteria in a predisposed subject (*Leçons du Mardi*, vol. 2, 347–53). Charcot noted that Klein had received help from "ses coréligionnaires" as well as the "association Israélite" in Metz during three years of wandering across Germany, England, Belgium, and France. On this point and elsewhere in his thesis, Meige added an anti-semitic tone, not present in Charcot's clinical remarks, to aspects of Jewish behavior, language, dress, and social assistance. The thesis was widely reviewed in the medical and lay

press, including Drumont's *La Libre Parole* and the Jewish press. See Goldstein, "The Wandering Jew." One of the favorable reviews came from Meige's friend, Jean-Baptiste Charcot, who served as his father's last intern in 1893. *Archives de Neurologie* 26 (1893): 343–46. Charcot's abrupt death one month after presiding over Meige's thesis seems to have halted the impetus for this vein of research at the Salpêtrière. Meige had referred to a forthcoming "étude sur *la pathologie des Juifs* où la question sera traitée dans son ensemble" to be published by A. Dutil, Charcot's current chef de clinique, but Dutil's synthesis never appeared.

80. "Je me suis cependant levé vers 6 heures du matin reveillé par toutes sortes de cris provenant du marché de Tetuan. Nous voilà en pleine féerie. C'est un vrai conte des mille et une nuits réalisé. Rien ne choque: tout est exotique et pure" (Letter, August 10. Added to Jeanne's letter of Wednesday).

81. "l'Afrique, l'Afrique vraie. Comme hier – les chênes-lièges, les palmiers noirs, les lauriers rose quand il y a un ruisseau, etc. etc. – vraie vérité enfin" (ibid.).

82. "Adieu fille de Grenade, nous allons bientôt rendre à ta mère une pieuse visit : . . . c'est que Tetuan c'est Grenade et Grenade c'est Tetuan."

83. The identification of Tetuan with Granada, a commonplace observation by European travelers, is nonetheless particularly strong in Charcot's hereditary metaphor. That the neurologist's search for a presumed unifying model underlying diverse "formes frustes" went beyond intellectual needs is suggested by his account of his discovery of the *type forme* of major hysteria: "Je n'y voyais absolument que confusion, et l'impuissance à laquelle j'étais réduit me causait une certaine irritation ; lorsqu'un jour, par une sorte d'intuition je me suis dit: mais c'est toujours la même chose ; alors j'en conclus qu'il y avait là une maladie particulière, l'hystéria major . . . " (*Leçons du mardi*, 7 février 1888, vol. 1, 174).

84. Freud, "Charcot," 12. Freud states that the description of Charcot as a "visuel" came from Charcot's own characterization of himself.

85. See Gelfand, "Charcot's Brains," *Brain and Language*, 69 (1999): 31–55, esp. 43–46.

86. On receiving long-awaited news by telegraph from his wife, Charcot ruminated on the role of subjectivity in altering perception but he stopped well short of rejecting the sensations as primary and necessary: "Le ciel de Tetuan nous en parait plus beau, l'air plus léger, la chaleur moindre, et tout ce que l'on voit plus transparent. Ce que c'est que de nous et comme ils ont raison ceux qui disent que tout est en nous . . . à la condition toutefois qu'il vienne q[uel]q[ue] chose du dehors, bien entendu!! " (**A, 6 c-d**).

87. For example: "one of the most beautiful landscapes that can be imagined: the town of Ceuta, enclosed by walls ending in the jetty, emerges against the background of the blue sea, like a small map in relief, and in the distance, Gibraltar" (**B, 4-a**).

88. "*L'accumulation de tombes blanches fait – au loin l'*effet *de linge blanches qu'on sèche en plein air*" (**A, 12-d**).

89. "*L'air d'un grand benêt,*" "*L'air d'un sacristain de synagogue*" (**A, 4-b, 4-c**).

90. Charcot also conveys the visual with forms of "*regarder,*" "*apercevoir,*" "*présenter,*" and "*apparaître.*"

91. "*Entendre*" occurs nine times, but "*oreille*" not at all, while "*œil*" or "*yeux*" come into play ten times as means of perception.

92. "*C'est une perfection, un paradis au point de la vision et de l'odorat.*"

93. "*Une empreinte visuelle difficile à effacer*" (**A, 11-b**).

94. "*Tout cela me revient à l'esprit en faisant mon croquis . . . je prendrais bien encore un croquis . . .*"

95. "*Que l'âge commence à émonder chez moi la vivacité des impressions neuves, je dois dire que j'ai été profondément remué par tout cela . . .*" (*Letter of Wednesday* [August 10, Tetuan]).

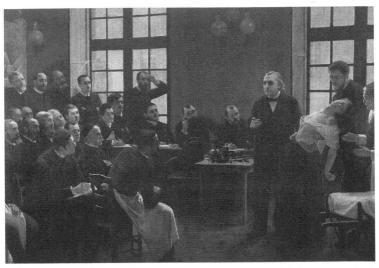

Fig. 1: Group portrait, *A Clinical Lesson at the Salpêtrière* by André Brouillet. Painting, 1887. Engraving, 1889.

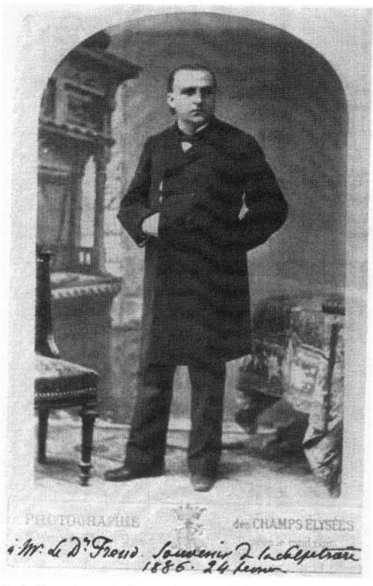

Fig. 2: Charcot's portrait photograph, autographed to "M. le docteur Freud." [*Dated February 24, 1886, the day Freud departed the Salpêtrière.*]

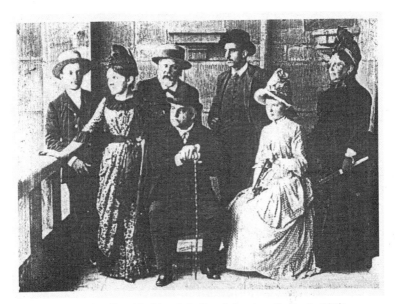

Fig. 3: Charcot family with friends in San Sebastian, Spain, in 1887. [*Charcot is seated in front, his daughter, Jeanne, standing to his right and son, Jean-Baptiste, to his left. Philippe Burty stands behind Charcot.*] Source: Charcot family papers.

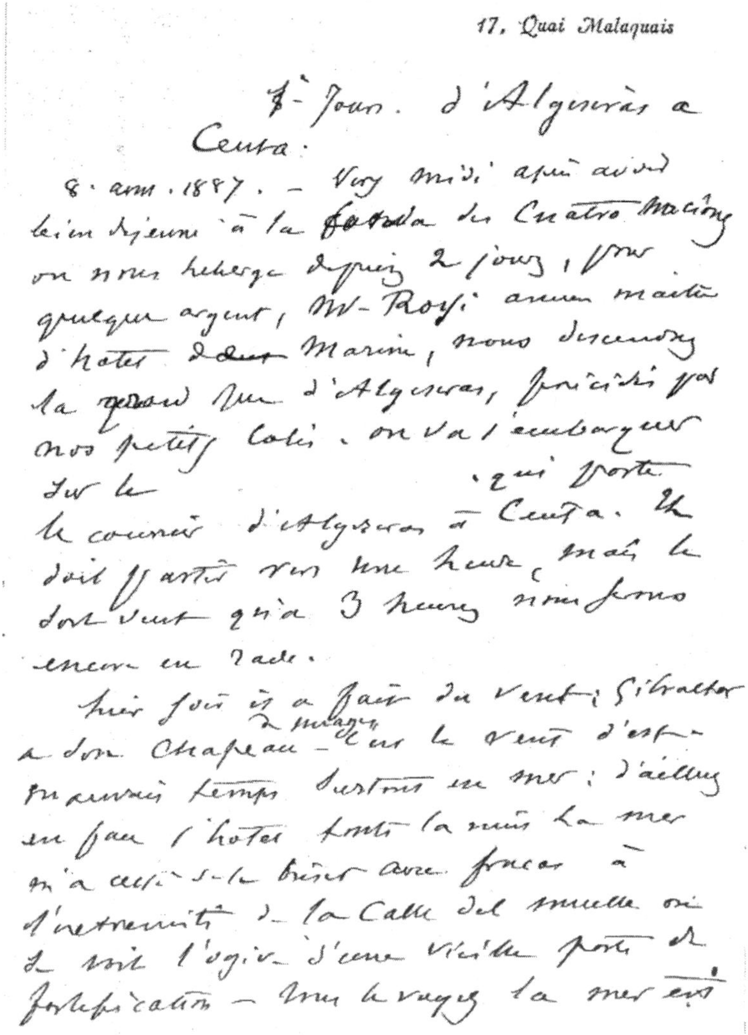
17, Quai Malaquais

1er Jour. d'Algesiras a Ceuta.

8 août 1887. — Vers midi après avoir bien déjeuné à la Fonda des Cuatro Naciones où nous héberge depuis 2 jours, pour quelque argent, M. Rossi ancien maître d'hôtel ~~de la~~ Marine, nous descendons la ~~grand~~ rue d'Algesiras, précédés par nos petits colis. On va s'embarquer sur le   qui porte le courrier d'Algesiras à Ceuta. Il doit partir vers une heure, mais le dort vent qu'à 3 heures nous sommes encore en rade.

Hier soir il a fait du vent; Gibraltar a son chapeau de nuages — c'est le vent d'est — mauvais temps surtout en mer; d'ailleurs en face l'hôtel toute la nuit la mer s'a acc... se briser avec fracas à l'extrémité de la Calle del muelle où se voit l'ogive d'une vieille porte de fortification — sous les vagues la mer est

Fig. 4: First page of Moroccan journal.
[***"First day. From Algeciras to Ceuta, August 8, 1887."***]

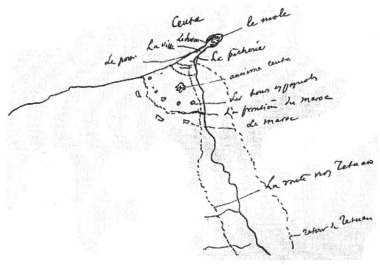

Fig. 5: Charcot's hand-drawn plan of Ceuta indicating sights visited.
Source: Charcot family papers.

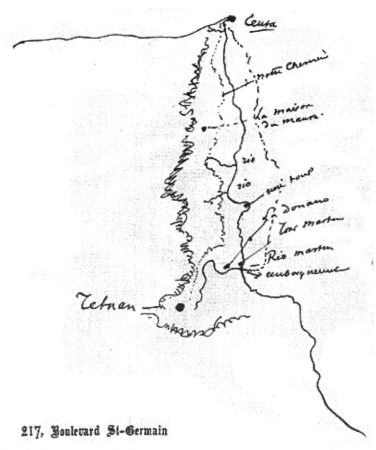

Fig. 6: Charcot's sketch of his party's route to Tetuan by land and return by sea. Source: Charcot family papers.

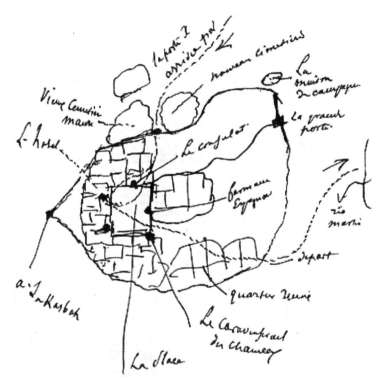

Fig. 7: Charcot's hand-drawn plan of Tetuan with locations indicated.
Source: Charcot family papers.

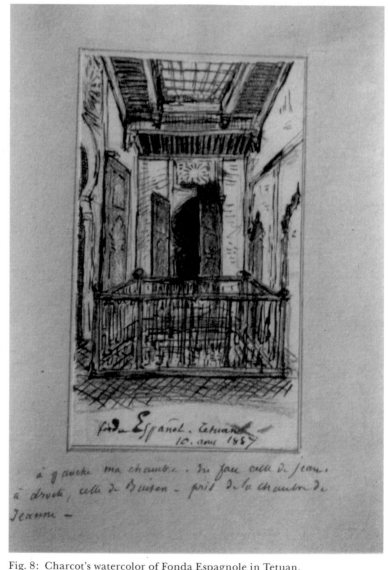

Fig. 8: Charcot's watercolor of Fonda Espagnole in Tetuan.
[*Labelled by Charcot: "The Spanish Inn, Tetuan, August 10, 1887. On the left, my room. Facing, Jean's, to the right, Buison's. Drawn from Jeanne's room."*]
Source: Charcot family papers.

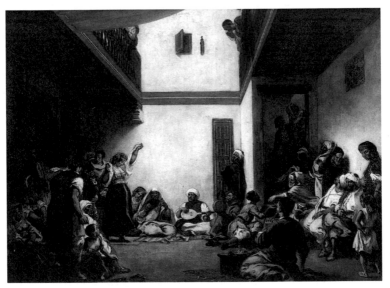

Fig. 9: Eugène Delacroix: *Noce Juive dans le Maroc.*
Source: Wikipedia Commons. Le Louvre, Paris.

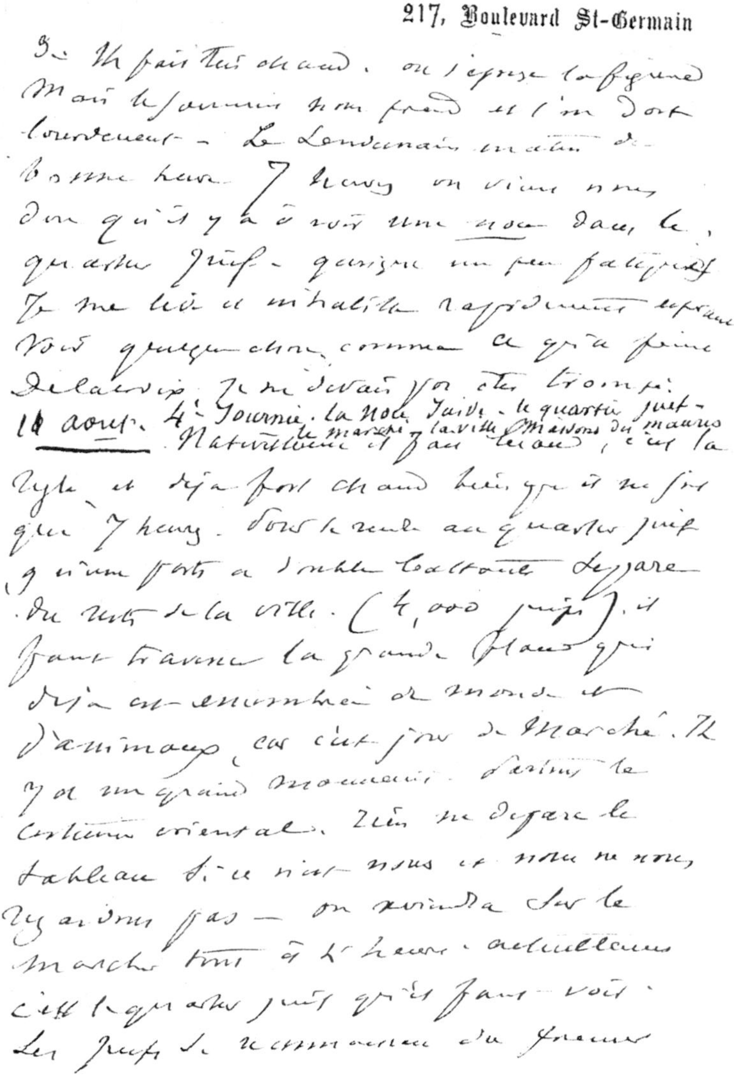

[handwritten French manuscript, largely illegible cursive]

... Il fait très chaud ...

11 août. 4e Journée. la Noce Juive ...

Fig. 10: "4th day August 11: The Jewish Wedding" Moroccan journal.

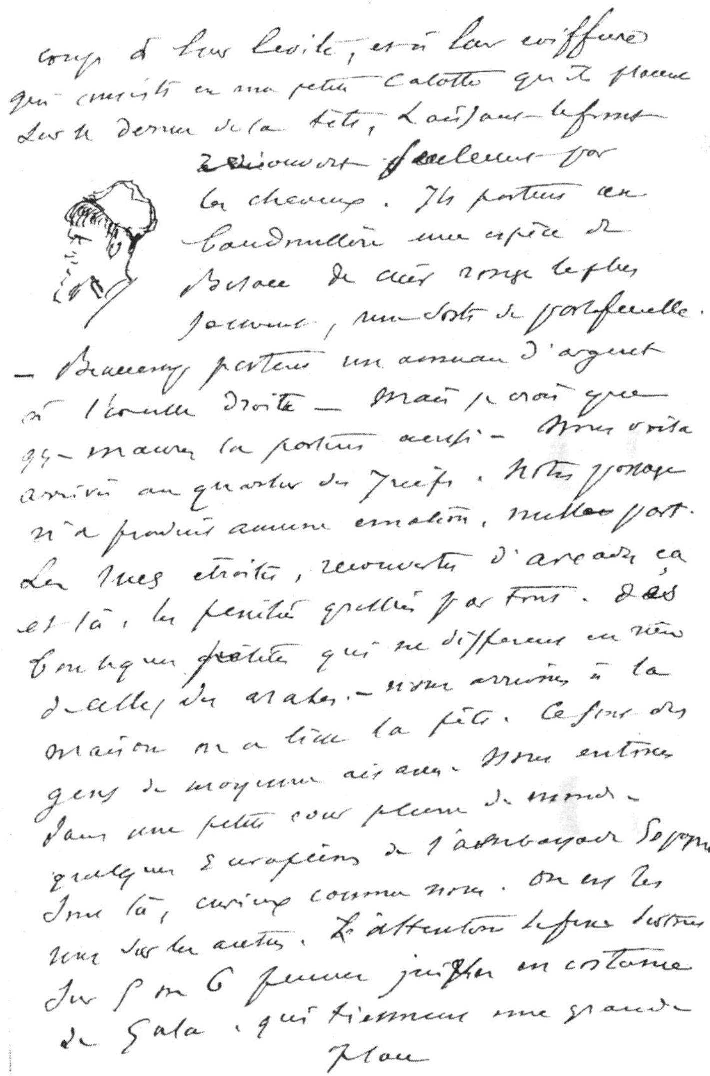

corps de leur Lévite, et à leur coiffure
qui consiste en une petite calotte qu'ils placent
sur le derrière de la tête, laissant le front
découvert seulement par
les cheveux. Ils portent en
bandoulière une espèce de
besace de cuir rouge le plus
souvent, une sorte de portefeuille.
— Beaucoup portent un anneau d'argent
à l'oreille droite — Mais je crois que
qq-maures la portent aussi — Nous voilà
arrivés au quartier des Juifs. Notre passage
n'a produit aucune émotion, nulle part.
Les rues étroites, recouvertes d'arcades ça
et là, les fenêtres grillées partout. Des
boutiques petites qui ne diffèrent en rien
de celles des arabes. — Nous arrivons à la
maison où a lieu la fête. Ce sont des
gens de moyenne aisance. Nous entrons
dans une petite cour pleine de monde —
quelques Européens de l'ambassade Espagnole,
sont là, curieux comme nous. On est les
uns sur les autres. L'attention se porte surtout
sur 5 ou 6 femmes juives en costume
de Gala, qui tiennent une grande
place

Fig. 11: Charcot's sketch of a Jew. [***"their head covering which consists of a small cap worn on the back of the head, leaving the forehead covered just by the hair"***], Moroccan journal.

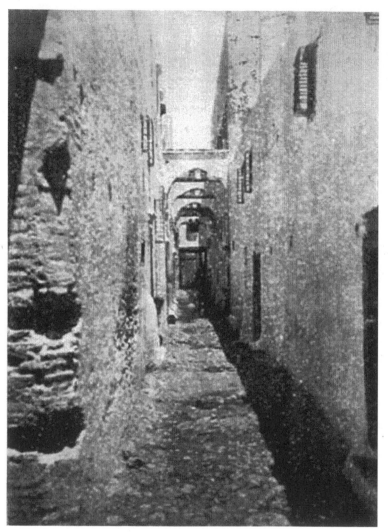

Fig. 12: Photograph purchased by Charcot of a street in the Jewish quarter of Tetuan. Source: Charcot family papers.

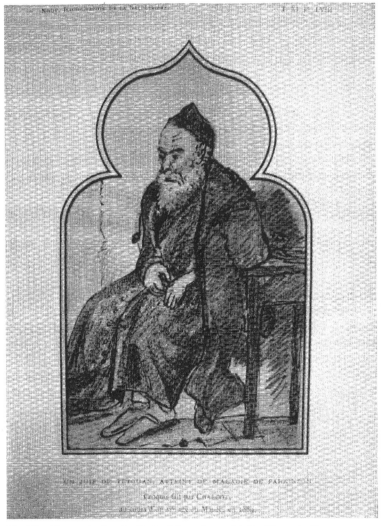

Fig. 13: Charcot's sketch of a Jewish patient with Parkinson's disease.
Source: Henry Meige, "Charcot artiste," *Nouvelle iconographie de la Salpêtrière* 11 (1898), plate 58, between pp. 498–99. [*Meige identifies Charcot's sketch of the Tetuan Jew as having been done during a Moroccan trip "in 1889" [sic]*]

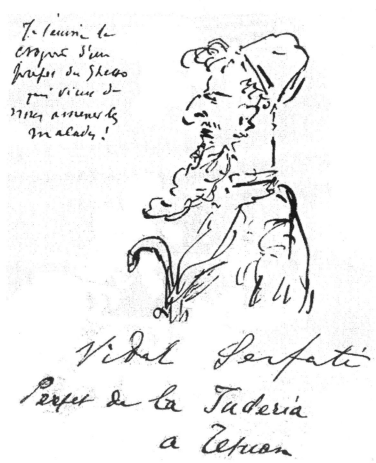

Fig. 14: Charcot's sketch of a Jewish leader of Tetuan. [*Charcot identified this crude representation as "Vidal Serfati, Prefect of Judea." His note to Mme Charcot reads: "I send you the sketch of a prefect of the ghetto who has just brought the patients to us!"*] Source: Charcot family papers.

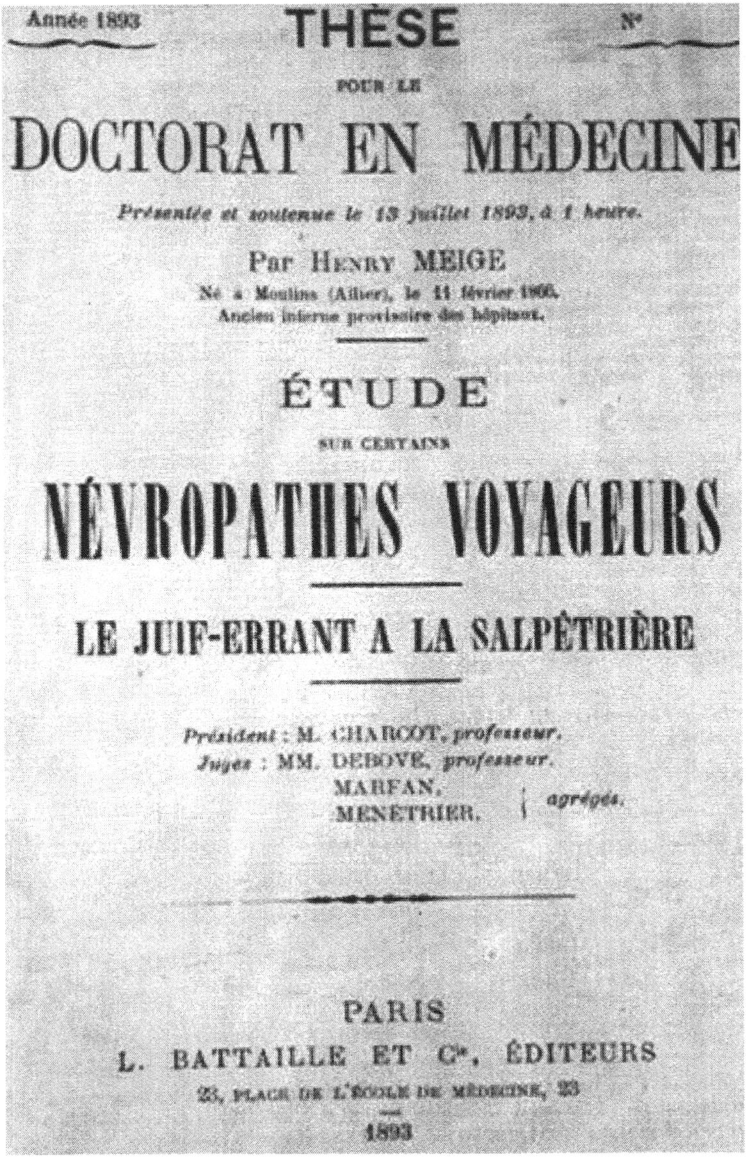

Année 1893   **THÈSE**   Nᵒ

POUR LE

DOCTORAT EN MÉDECINE

Présentée et soutenue le 13 juillet 1893, à 1 heure.

Par Henry MEIGE

Né à Moulins (Allier), le 11 février 1866,
Ancien interne provisoire des hôpitaux.

ÉTUDE

SUR CERTAINS

NÉVROPATHES VOYAGEURS

LE JUIF-ERRANT A LA SALPÊTRIÈRE

Président : M. CHARCOT, *professeur.*
Juges : MM. DEBOVE, *professeur.*
MARFAN,
MÉNÉTRIER. } *agrégés.*

PARIS

L. BATTAILLE ET Cⁱᵉ, ÉDITEURS

23, PLACE DE L'ÉCOLE DE MÉDECINE, 23

1893

Fig. 15: Title page of Henry Meige, "A study of certain neurotic travelers. The Wandering Jew at the Salpêtrière." [*Paris medical thesis, 1893, presided over by Charcot.*] Source: Copy in Bibliothèque Charcot, Paris.

II

English Translation

Eight days in Morocco. Ceuta and Tetuan

[1-a] 1st day from Algeciras to Ceuta.

8 August 1887.—Toward noon, after a good meal at the inn of the Quatro Naciones, where, for the past 2 days, we have lodged for a certain sum with M. Royi, a retired steward in the navy, we walk down the main street of Algeciras trailing our small parcels. We're going to embark on the [blank in text] which carries the mail from Algeciras to Ceuta. It was to leave around one o'clock, but fate decreed that at 3, we would still be in the harbor.

Last evening, the wind howled; Gibraltar is wearing its cap of clouds,—it's the east wind—bad weather, especially at sea: what is more, the whole night long, the sea never stopped crashing furiously against the *calle del muelle*[1] across from the inn from which one can see the arch of an old fortification. "The sea is **[1-b]** a bit rough in the gulf, what will it be like in the strait? I would not embark at this moment; I would wait from 3 to 7 days counting before setting out. And, in any case, what is there to do in Ceuta? The inns are disgusting. I was rather poorly accommodated there; I arrived in the evening and left the following morning without seeing anything. And then, Tetuan . . . but that's not very certain." Thus, did our young consul[2] voice his opinion yesterday and, while he was speaking, I saw our friend B[urty][3] go pale, his features stiffen . . . I thought he was experiencing some kind of malaise! Yes, he was in pain, but his suffering was in his mind [*moralement*]. The closing words of the consul had changed his mind and, before I went to bed, Buison,[4] with a diplomatic look, conveyed to me the following: "I have the delicate task of informing you that B[urty] will not come with us tomorrow." "How come, bah, why?" "He asked me to beg you not to insist . . ." "All right, I won't insist."

And that is why the next morning, [1-c] four of us, instead of five, stepped down into the boat which was to take us to the Correo. Farewell Burty, farewell Arène . . . at least have a good time and write to my wife every day.

Buison went out of his way for us. We received letters for the director of the prison of Ceuta, for the governor, for all the authorities more or less; and the governor of Algeciras personally promised that the military telegraph would operate for our benefit, if we needed it and if it was possible. In this way he nicely reattached us to Europe by a Hope.

So here we are on our way, after 2 hours waiting. Are they waiting for the mail? Why is the mail 2 hours late? . . . a Spanish thing. At last we depart; a bit rough, but none of us feels out of sorts, not even Buison, who was afraid. Poor Burty, he could have done it, for here we are in sight of Ceuta . . . but alas! Gibraltar's cap was to play a nasty trick.

[1-d] It is 6 o'clock. We are more than two hours late. The people who were to wait for our skiff [*barque*] must have given up. We get down into the skiff where we're rather tightly

packed; unconsciously I wrinkle my brow slightly . . . arrival messed up, I whisper to myself . . . I am wrong. Everything is fine, for as we draw near to the port, we make out about ten people who clearly are waiting for us. Among them, distinguished by his height and dress, is the director of the prison, an excellent man, tall, thin, very helpful, wearing an absurd cravat and an endlessly long white jacket which nicely throws into relief his Don Quixote-like form. Also there, at last, is Bajonna[5] who was to serve as our guide and protector [*providence*] for the expedition to Tetuan. Our small parcels are unloaded. They number 7, and are immediately grasped by as many men of rather sinister appearance who seem to be under the direction of an 8th man of the same appearance. They are the galley convicts, we learn en route, "But you can be assured of your safety." That's fine. Forward march.

[**2-a**] In addition, we noticed a tall old Jew wearing the Oriental Jewish robe [*lévite*]. "Come with me," he said to me: "I am the guide for the Spanish inn. You will need me."— The Jew gave me the impression, I don't why, that he ought to be named Aaron . . . And, indeed, that is his name.

Our arrival caused a stir in the town. Everyone looked at us. "Who are these eccentrics [*originaux*] who are coming to see the country at this time of year[6]—they are crazy . . . English, English." "No, not English," we say, "but French. And we are not as crazy as you think." They will come to see that. On the way, we meet a crowd of Jews and, as well, a crowd of Moors of all kinds: peasants, bourgeoisie, merchants, black and white Moroccans. Several are pushing donkeys loaded with all sorts of things. Here we are already in Moroccan country. Yes, a good third of the way, perhaps.

[**2-b**] We come to a rather poor-looking house; it faces the large emplacement where the soldiers of the Spanish line get some fresh air. It's the Spanish inn; only there did they find

a place to lodge us. War is war [*à la guerre, comme à la guerre*]; we are not here to amuse ourselves. Putting up with all the vermin in creation is part of the programme. Besides, how can we be pitied, occupying the main apartment in the house, in disagreeably close contact with the proprietors? When nature calls in her special way we have to cross through their bedroom with three people in it, as well as the kitchen where a servant lives. When you have traversed all that, you are rewarded for your efforts with a picturesque set-up in the open air.

All that is just details; we dine, in short, not too badly and, in the evening, we welcome, at coffee time, our new friends of Ceuta [**2-c**] who have come to arrange tomorrow's excursions with us. However, it is getting late and I'm going to bed. Sleep comes quickly despite the fierce heat, the vague fear of insects, and the resounding noise from the piano of Mlle. X who, across the way, favors us with a few tunes from the à la mode Madrid play, the Gran via.[7]

2nd day. The fishery and the border of Morocco. [**fig. 5**]
The penal colony.
9 August 1887. From father to son, going back countless centuries, the great fisheries of Almadrade (?)[8] have been in the hands of the Bayonna family. Their son escorts us there this morning. We leave Ceuta on the south-east side, and find ourselves on the sea coast, under the rampart. We are in a kind of warehouse in which a huge quantity of fish, dried-out flying fish especially, are hanging. This is the depot under the supervision of Bayonna senior, an old man of 65, all shriveled and wrinkled like an old apple, but still fresh enough, although his stomach bothers him. But it is the fishing itself that has to be seen. Great nets are placed at perhaps a kilometer from the beach. Over there, we can make out the boats carrying them and the fishermen who are going to lift them up right away. We

head for the spot. The sea is a bit rough, and one of our fellows, who performs this task frequently in an effort *to get used to it*,[9] soon gets sea sick . . . his unfortunate courage does him credit! Here we are near the great nets: at a given signal the circle of boats closes. At the same time, each boat pulls up its catch; the circle tightens rapidly, and the poor creatures, hundreds of them, mostly flying fish, thrash about noisily as they strike against one another, displaying in turn their steel backs and their silver bellies. A few, straightening up like springs, manage to jump overboard . . . good luck. But, for the others, no more hope . . . *Lasciate ogni speranza*,[10] the breath of life in these poor creatures expires with their effort **[ms B][3-a]**. Everywhere, just convulsions and death agony. All that suffering and death, it is dreadful; but such is the law. Nature knows no morality, and the big eat the little or the other way round.

We return to the inn and we go over to the side along the jetty for a visit to the penal colony. The colony is really everywhere in the town because the majority of the convicts [*galériens*] circulate under the surveillance of sorts of warders who are distinguishable only by a stripe. But they all live in the prison and, if you want to see them, that is where you must go to find those who never leave and those who are punished in chains. The institution is as one might imagine: large common sleeping rooms, pitiful and fetid, dreadful courtyards.

[3-b] Among the inmates several rascals *di primo cartello*,[11] who looked like butter wouldn't melt in their mouths,[12] are pointed out to us. They wear a gray shirt and cloth trousers of the same color, nothing bright or green, just like our penal colonies of old. We soon have our fill of this inspection. Besides it is very hot. We're thirsty and hungry. We return to the inn via a long narrow street where the buildings resemble those of Algeciras, the small window with a grill on the ground floor, convenient for lovers. On the way we pass

Moors, Jews, and convicts—but we have already encountered all three.

The second part of the day will be used to good purpose. It is devoted to [3-c] the excursion called the *Serai*,[13] Ceuta fashion. All our friends will accompany us on horseback or by mule. Jeanne, myself and Buison will be driven a certain distance in a carriage, the governor's own, after which we will have to mount a mule or horse for close to an hour.

It is around 3 o'clock; we have let the hottest part of the day go by. However it remains so hot that I forgo the niceties. I leave aside cravat and collar; I wear an unstarched shirt, no jacket, and, for underclothes, my thin silk which I often use as a bathrobe. This abandon seems justified by the consideration that, excepting Jeanne, there are no women with us . . . But alas! There will be *women* . . . shortly [3-d]. So we depart. We will cross the three fortified walls which protect Ceuta on the Moroccan side . . . fortifications dating from the 17th century at least, good at best against the Moroccans. We enter the countryside.

The land rises gradually on the right-hand side, and to the left is the sea, for we are on a narrow peninsula. A series of hills are in front of us and, in the background, the true mountains, high and looking somber. On the right, I am shown Old Ceuta (Roman?) where there are ancient murals and where they have found mosaics. Here and there are a few country houses. On the left, a small mosque which seems well kept up. Moors come and go on the road and mix with Spaniards. We advance and, on the left, we [4-a] perceive a large square building which is a fort and barracks. There we call a halt and leave the carriage for the mules. But before climbing down, I turn around to see one of the most beautiful landscapes that can be imagined: the town of Ceuta, enclosed by walls ending in the jetty, emerges against the background of the blue sea, like a small map in relief, and in the distance, Gibraltar.

It's time to dismount. Alas, there are ladies in blue silk dresses with frills and flounces, and very fine-looking military men who appear in front of us. [?] Where can I hide? If I had known . . . etc. My lord, so much the worse; I will perhaps not be noticed in the midst [4-b] of all the fine horsemen who are with me. But I am introduced as someone who is a personage!!!!! I put on the best face possible, avoiding the ladies' stares as best I can.[14]

It is time to leave. They sit Jeanne and me on a mule. They hoist me up on a kind of chair [*cacolet*] where I arrange myself like someone disabled . . . which I am. I'm not too uncomfortable up there and I'm not upset with the experience since tomorrow I'll have to do this trick during 12 or 14 hours. Today's promenade by mule is going to take around 2 ½ hours; I multiply that figure by seven . . . and [4-c] after thinking about it, I conclude: it will be hard, but I can do it.

After the barracks post, the road stops. It becomes nothing more than a mule path. We go upward, always climbing. We go round one of the Spanish towers, with vertical stripes in rows that can be seen from Ceuta at separate intervals indicating the border of Morocco. Within there are soldiers who cannot be enjoying themselves much as time drags on, for the site is at once deserted, imposing and rather sad. Facing us are the mountains of Morocco, dark and somber and that is where we are heading. The yellow dog accompanying us, which looks like a greyhound and which I took to be an African dog, is, however, just a Spanish hunting dog. He causes some partridges to take flight here and there [4-d]. This delights most of our fellow travelers who, alas, remain in a philosophical and moral state of mind where that bloody sport, known as hunting, is considered a game of pleasure. As I indulge these thoughts, a small somber valley opens up in front of us where a tiny stream flows, separating the Spanish territory from Morocco. In the background are oleanders [*lauriers roses*] all in bloom. But on the other side, facing us, there is a dark green mountain with layers of superb cork oaks with dark leaves. It is imposing and a bit sad. At the top [illegible word] there is a small well-appointed square white house where, from afar, animals can be seen. That is where we are going.

The stream is crossed. Here we are in Morocco. No one but us on either side [5-a]. We experience a slight emotion of apprehension, completely instinctive, since there is absolutely nothing to fear. Yesterday, at Ceuta, where he had business, we met the chief of the station toward which we are heading. He has made our arrival known to his elder son who is replacing him in his absence. He is awaiting us ready to show us all the respect due to our status.

We confidently make our way up the hill by a zigzag foot-path; the little square white fort grows bigger as we approach and still we see no one. At last 2 human figures become visible against the white background of the square house. I don't like the look of them. One carries a net. They are dressed in mantles of a dirty grey color. We [5-b] keep climbing. We dismount, we have arrived. A few men take charge of our mules, and we slowly enter the enclosure of the poor fort. After crossing a courtyard, we are shown into a small room where we find the son of the chief, a young man of about 18, distinguished looking, a fez on his head. He gets up to welcome us with every politeness, extending his hand graciously. His young brother, 12 years old, is in a corner. The other people are soldiers of the post. We squat on cushions, seated around a tray on which there are coffee cups which seem to me to come from the rue de Paradis.[15] The teapot is more original, especially the small red lacquered box from which [5-c] a servant takes the tea. For we are to be offered a cup of tea and cake. What am I saying, a cup of tea? One must take 3 cups, more if desired—never less! This is considered polite, and we do as required, all the more willingly as this aromatic tea, which we will meet again in Tetuan, seems excellent to us in this insufferable heat........I would indeed have taken a 4th cup, but it is getting late. The day is waning, we must return to Ceuta. Besides, the conversation is languishing even though everyone here speaks a little Spanish. They say farewell cordially and hoist us up on our mules and away we go on the route by which we came. The sun rapidly sets, and when we arrive at Ceuta, it is night. We dine [5-d] heartily and go off to bed to sleep soundly [*à poings fermés*], as rapidly and deeply as possible, for tomorrow, we must get up at 5 o'clock and the journey will be rough.

3rd day.
From Ceuta to Tetuan [**fig. 6**]
—The Moor's house
—The gate of Tetuan locked
10 August 1887
The original plan had been to travel to Ceuta by sea, and Bayonna was to take us on his boat. But the wind was not favorable. In that kind of weather, one knows when one departs . . . but not when one arrives: could we cross the sand bar of the rio Martin? Etc. etc.

[6-a] These doubts were expressed. Certainly, it was added, there was no danger involved. If we do not get there, we will turn around. All these concerns did not appear to me to argue in favor of the sea crossing. By that route, if successful, we would gain the advantage of being on horseback only 2 or 3 hours; but we would risk perhaps losing 1 or 2 days and, for Jean's sake,[16] we did not have time to waste.

Dry land [*le plancher des vaches*] is the surer way; it will be long, perhaps difficult, but in the end we will arrive for sure. This last option was taken and put into practice. We will return by sea if, at that time, the wind will turn favorable.

[**6-b**] It is five o'clock in the morning. In the street, the mules are waiting for us. 2 mules carry the baggage and provision . . . for one must eat and get dressed . . . even in Africa. Buison, Jean and Bayonna are each astride a mule. Jeanne and I are each seated in chairs on mules like handicapped people . . . speaking for myself, for Jeanne only has infirmities which are natural to her sex. 2 Spanish drivers and Moors of the King, not armed, accompany us. One of the latter, we realized along the way, is a fine fellow and a philosopher. There is also a big Negro, quite young, with a slightly alarmed look, shaved head, except for a tuft of hair [**6-c**] on his right temple. They say he is a bit dim and the son of a great dogon chieftain.[17] So we go our way through the streets of the town, and leave by the gate to the fields, as yesterday. But instead of going to the right, we head left, alongside the sea, which we never desert, during the entire duration of our journey. It is hot, but the sky is slightly overcast in places. Perhaps we will not be absolutely cooked. Besides everyone is comfortable, and my outfit today matches yesterday's exactly. So we go for 4 hours; after that, we call a halt at the Moor's house . . . It is about half way. There we will find shade and water. We will halt for lunch [**6-d**] and a bit of a siesta; then we will start out again cool and refreshed . . . Such is the plan . . . We shall see that it had to be slightly modified in a few respects. On the left, the sea, on the right, mountains rising in tiers and advancing or falling back in a way that restricts or widens the plain, a few small rivers to cross. Such is the lay of the land from Ceuta to Tetuan. Moreover, no roads to speak of. Footpaths scarcely traced out; no trees, more or less dense bushes, of varying heights, forming at times tiny

woods in miniature. (Oleanders when we come to a river). No villages, this is the desert. A few fields of maize outside Tetuan. In the distance, half-way up, on the mountain a few huts for men who sift the wheat. And that is [7-a] the only trace of humanity that we see during the first 4 or 5 hours; nearly all that we see during the remaining 5 or 6 hours.

Soon we reach the 1st Moroccan doorway, a square house, which sits atop a high hill. Two Moors of the Emperor who are to accompany us emerge; one carries a gun, the other a bag. These 2 do not join in with our group. Sometimes they approach, then at other times they disappear—only to reappear a little afterwards at a turn in the way . . . they are definitely strange; as well they have a rather unhealthy look about them with their caped robes [*burnous*] that seem to be soaked with sweat [7-b].

We have been walking perhaps 2 hours when suddenly the plain widens out. In the middle we see a castle [*castillo*] in ruins covered with ivy—not far off, some stones are piled up in a way that marks off an oval shape of earth. It is a tomb. There are many others. On a few of the tombs, red rags hang from sticks planted in the ground, rags now faded which must have formerly had a beautiful red color. They mark the tomb of a chieftain, more or less canonized and elevated to the level of saint. It was here that the battle against the Moroccans took place which led to the march on Tetuan. More than 20 years ago, all that. The name Prim[18] returns to mind. We walk on and keep on walking. From time to time I look at [7-c] my watch. We're going to get to the Moor's place soon, no doubt! By this time hunger and thirst have set in. But where is this devil of a house of the Moor? We don't see it. Here are a few trees and rocks. We have lost sight of the sea. Anxiously, we walk on for nearly an hour: devil of a house gone astray. We begin to berate the Moors of the Emperor who led us down this wrong path. At last, there it is, a hut scarcely above the ground, hidden among the underbrush and tall cactus. The roof did not differ in color or shape from a few rocks lying here and there. The Moor opens the door—he's a man of 60 of rather distinguished [7-d] appearance, but poor in his [illegible word]. An adorable little girl of 5 or 6 is there with him; she is sulking but still stares at us very attentively with her little eyes black as a jaybird. She is his daughter and there lies a story: the mother and father got along badly with one another; she lives in Tetuan; he, the old man, prefers solitude over staying in town with his wife. In any case, it is of no concern to us—they say he is a man not without wealth. He seems to have come from a family of Granada and to have brought "his papers" which show him to be the owner of a house in Granada, etc. etc. Whatever may be, he lives here in a simple hut, around which is a small fruit garden. There are chickens.

[8-a] In the courtyard, a large fig tree provides a bit of shade, which we increase by stretching out a cloth overhead. We sit down there for lunch. And we are brought cool water. The plan thus is realized to the letter: we have had shade and water at the Moor's. I attempt a brief siesta, but I doze with one eye open. We don't have time to spare. The second part of the trip will be longer than the first. We must not arrive too late. We say our farewells to the Moor, to the little girl and are on our way.

We approach the sea again and we often have to cross streams, little rivers that are indicated from afar by the tiny oleanders nestled in their beds [8-b]. A few look deep: how can we cross? Bajonna, our guide, explains that their mouths are all silted up at this time of year—which we would have been able to guess by the absence of current and by wading in with our animals and seeing that the water barely reached as high as their bellies. So things in fact turned out, and we forded the "great river with dry feet."[19] Two hours pass; from

the head of the caravan, the cry is heard: water! water! [*aqua!
aqua!*] It's a well. We call a halt and drink a little; it is perhaps
3 o'clock. It is hot, we are thirsty. The well is deep, the water
low. A Moor goes down clinging to the stones. He re-emerges
[8-c] with a full jug and we drink the cool water, which is a bit
cloudy. I took shelter under a tall bush where, judging by the
debris of all kinds strewn over the ground, people had often
sat. I began to muse . . . here we are, far from Europe, from
France, from Paris, . . . here there's nothing commonplace
. . . places nearly unexplored. I was enjoying the sensation
imparted by the idea "of an unknown well where one is the
first to drink" as Lucretius says. Alas a piece of yellowed newspaper lies on the ground. It seems to have been used to hold
some food, unless it was for something else . . . I read in large
letters, *Le Figaro*!!! *July 23 literary supplement.* This supplement
isn't sold separately. July 23rd, and [8-d] we're August 10th. Only
17 days ago . . . *Le Figaro.* That's it all right. Alas! What a come
down . . . and how that reminds us to be modest. Yes, be modest and do not forget that it is *Le Figaro*, alas! which represents
us, especially in foreign lands . . . in the station of Charing
Cross, in all the patios of Seville, at Saint Petersburg, and in
the desert of Tetuan! I will take this dirty fragment and place
it in my scrapbook and I'll look at it from time to time . . . with
melancholy.[20]

I get up and rejoin the group drinking water, who are
sharing a watermelon. On the mound where they are sitting,
there is no more space. One of the Moors of the King noticed;
he goes up to my [9-a] son and, tapping him gently on the
shoulder, says to him, in Spanish, "Your father is not seated."
My son gets up and I sit down in his place. An example of Arab
manners that is in sum very edifying and which demonstrates
that, even if we are among the people of Barbary, we are not
with barbarians.

Once again, en route, the path gradually moves away from the sea which is soon lost to view. On the right, a small lake with a flock of wild birds. B. takes the gun from one of the Moors of the Emperor accompanying us. The shot is fired, the bird takes flight . . . and is not wounded. So much the better, I say to myself *in petto*. And there's one who can still enjoy for a long time his bird's life which **[9-b]** he undoubtedly values a lot. Bon voyage.[21]

It's six o'clock; we begin to wonder seriously about Tetuan. Where is it? It cannot be seen, it is hidden behind a mountain range, which rises to a kind of cape on the top of which sits a tower. Tetuan will remain hidden to us for a long time yet, but on the left we see a plain which extends to the sea. Not far off are two square white buildings, one larger than the other. The 2nd, nearer to us, is the customs house. The other, which seems to touch the sea is the Tour Martin. That is where we will embark to return to Ceuta, if the wind is favorable. We come to **[9-c]** a sort of farmhouse perched on a hill which we go around. Our Moors of the King have acquaintances there. They have gone up, we heard them chatting there . . . They come down on the run and soon catch up.

We go on, ever onward . . . when will we get there?

In an hour . . . more or less. At last, there are gardens enclosed by high bamboo walls. From time to time an open door permits a view of a country house; we hear voices in the garden. We begin to meet people on the road coming and going . . . most of them greet us and say a few words to our Moors. We're undoubtedly getting close . . . fortunately! For the sun is setting and we know from experience that night comes on quickly here. We must not **[9-d]** arrive after the gates are locked. As a precaution, we dispatch one of our Moors to the town. He takes off on the run and soon disappears behind one of those bamboo walls which enclose the country houses. The hoofs of our mules resound as they strike the ground. We're on a paved road, very poorly paved without a doubt and full of holes . . . But this must be a main road. We are getting close without a doubt. It's nearly dark. On the right, on a hill some strange and imposing structures are visible. We are told that it is the old Moorish cemetery; on the left, a wall about 2 meters high permits the view of the tops of small isolated structures, rather sinister looking, whose shape can't be discerned because of the darkness. It is the new Moorish cemetery.

[10-a] At last we perceive a large white wall with niches pierced by a great door—on top of which is a square window. Is the gate open or closed, I wonder, from the rear of the caravan where I am? Suddenly, we are stopped—therefore the gate is closed.[22] Are we going to sleep outside?—they knock and they talk, inside and outside . . . there seem to be problems. Suddenly the shutter of the little square window over the door flies open with a bang, a light appears, then the silhouette of a man; a shrill voice articulates something which seems to me not at all favorable to our cause: "Christian dogs . . . go sleep in the open air,"[23] [10-b] or something similar without a doubt . . . definitely it is going badly. However, a good bed would really suit me after this hard day . . . A moment of silence. Suddenly the gate opens and here we are, inside . . . we had connections in the place . . . The Moor had arrived in time and a few *taffetas* had resolved the difficulties.

Here we are on a paved street, narrow, can't see a thing—but, after a few paces, on the right, a big open door lets us see a vast room lit up by numerous lamps. It is a mosque. We keep moving on down the narrow resounding streets in nearly complete obscurity, rarely meeting a passer-by from time to time.

[10-c] We emerge on a large square, empty at the moment . . . again a mosque, open and brightly lit. We go back into the shadows of the small narrow streets—here we are in an alley.

Suddenly the head of the caravan stops. A small hunched-back Moor, named Tach Tach, with whom we shall later have ample acquaintance, shines his lantern on us. We leave our mounts and enter through a single small door. As soon as this is passed, we enter the patio of a Moorish house . . . it is the Spanish inn [**fig. 8**].

Yes, we will get to know it better tomorrow. This is indeed the house of a Moor of middling wealth [*moyenne aisance*]. Nothing in the construction has been altered: around the patio are 4 or 5 rooms [*cuartos*] without windows. One will be our dining room.

[**10-d**] The large doors have been removed from the 4 *cuartos* on the first floor, also without windows. The only light that can get in comes from small loopholes above the large green double door with cube-shaped hinges, that are seen everywhere here. These doors are closed from the inside with the help of an enormous, very primitive bolt. On one of the shutters of the large door, there is a smaller door which can be opened by itself at night. One wonders where the daylight will come from tomorrow morning. But, looking upward, I perceive the dark sky with bright stars in constellations. The ceiling is pierced in the *azotia*.[24] That is how light comes in and rain too, and that explains why a sort of basin [*impluvium*] has been built on the ground of the patio—yes, everything is Moorish here . . . down to [**11-a**] the cut of the doors which lead from the patio to the first floor and one which leads from the first floor to the *azotia*. The door which goes from the patio to the corridor leading to the street has the same indentations. Only the Arab furniture is missing, replaced by good heavy Spanish furniture. Thus we will have beds, commodes, chests, etc. etc., chairs, arm-chairs, and we will not be obliged to squat in oriental fashion while eating or receiving visitors . . . which would be for me devilishly uncomfortable given the rigidity of my lower limbs.

Dinner is ready. We meet Madame Juanna, a beautiful Spanish specimen,[25] dark and well-endowed; also **[11-b]** very friendly is Juan, the innkeeper, her husband, a fine man, and the Jewish servants who go to great lengths to please us. Lastly is the small Moor, Tach Tach, who from now on, hobbling along [*clopin clopant*], equipped with a big staff and a gun, and a lantern at night, will lead us in our wanderings through the town . . . an ambiguous fellow, a bit mysterious, hesitating between this and that [*ménageant la chèvre et les choux*], and serving as liaison between Israel, Mohammed and the Pope . . . a great diplomat at heart as far as I can tell . . . I'll think about it. A good little trip to Tetuan in the hot season . . . why not? We're tired and go to sleep. Serious business can wait till tomorrow.

[Ms A] [3-a] It's very hot. I sponge my face. But sleep takes hold and I sleep deeply. The next morning, at the early hour of 7, they let us know that we can see a *marriage* in the Jewish quarter. Although a bit tired, I get up and dress quickly, hoping to see something like what Delacroix painted. I was not to be disappointed.

August 11 4th day. The Jewish wedding—the Jewish quarter—the town market—Moorish houses. **[figs. 9 and 10]**
Naturally, the weather is beautiful and already quite hot. That's the rule here although it is only 7 o'clock. To get to the Jewish quarter (4,000 Jews), which is separated from the rest of the town by a gate with a double door, one must cross the main square, already filled with people and livestock, for today is market day. There is much milling about with oriental costumes everywhere. Nothing detracts from the picture [*le tableau*] except us, and we don't look at ourselves. We will come back to the market shortly but, for now, it's the Jewish quarter which must be seen.

The Jews are recognizable right away [3-b] by their robe [*lévite*] and by their head covering which consists of a small cap worn on the back of the head, leaving the forehead covered just by the hair [**fig. 11**]. In a shoulder strap [*bandoulière*], they carry a kind of sac, most often of red leather, a sort of money bag. Many wear a silver ring on the right ear. But I believe a few Moors wear that as well.

We arrive in the Jewish quarter [**fig. 12**]. Our passing through caused no stir anywhere. Narrow streets, covered over by arcades here and there, grills over the windows everywhere, shops with grills just like those of the Arabs. We arrive at the house where the celebration is to take place. These are folks of middling wealth. We enter a small courtyard filled with people. A few Europeans from the Spanish embassy are there, curious like us. We are one on top of the other. Attention is riveted especially on 5 or 6 Jewish women in festive attire who occupy a large place, [3-c] caps of velvet on their heads, gilded embroidered fringes, enormous earrings—hair replaced by a black wig. The eyes are beautiful, in general, but the face is often puffy and scrofulous—a vest, recalling somewhat those of Toreadors, in dark green or dark blue velvet, with embroideries, a wide, thick, weighty skirt, in velvet of the same color, with huge embroideries on one corner. The skirt is open in the middle. The women wear necklaces, rich in appearance, bearing the two-headed eagle of the house of Austria. An old rabbi who is there and passes, perhaps legitimately, for a scholar wears the same costume as the Jews wore 300 years ago when they lived in Castille. The Jews of Tetuan were indeed Jews coming from Castille who had been hounded into exile. They all speak Spanish, a rather pure form, so it is said. Thus they would appear to have no bitterness toward their persecutors since they have kept their dress (?), their language, and even the eagle!!!! But we must pass from the courtyard [3-d] into the house where interesting things are going on. We enter a small room also jammed with people. But they offer space to the Europeans. They move aside to let them pass. The heat is suffocating, and it baffles me how those unfortunate beings in their heavy thick festive attire can withstand such heat. Really they seem oblivious to it and remain rather *pale*. The room we enter is quite small. Here again, there are ten seated women, richly attired, of varying age, but, on the whole, rather young, occupying an enormous space. But our attention is focused on the bride who is seated, motionless in a corner surrounded by 5 [illegible word] women, including her mother. She along with another woman prepare the bride's coiffure. They put on a sort of diadem; the other parts of the costume have already been arranged, one by one, doubtless with ceremony comparable to that observed for arranging the coiffure. The latter consists of a sort of rolled up diadem around the head, which must be very hot. At this point the black wig has already been substituted for the natural hair!

[4-a] The pins are put in place slowly, during which time the women chant monotonously to the steady rhythm of a Basque drum. They are interrupted from time to time by a sort of modulated plaintive groaning by another woman. (She seems to me to be a servant). The overall effect is powerful and penetrating. One feels transported back centuries in time, creating the sensation of a dream.

But let's come back to the bride. During this long torture, she remains completely motionless—one could say she has a face of wax. Her eyes are closed. Doubtless, no expression ought to adorn the lightly made-up face on which beauty marks [*mouches*] have been placed here and there. It is painful to see the unfortunate happy person. What would she do if she becomes hot or if her nose starts to itch? Suffer? Would she be disowned for scratching [4-b] her nose? At last, the ritual of dressing the bride is finished. She rises to her feet and takes a few steps in the room where she has been dressed and where the nuptial bed is. I notice that she is short and is wearing high heels.—in comes the groom who looks like a big fool and who, incongruously, in my view, wears a European suit[26]—cloth overcoat, top hat on his head, white veil on his shoulders,[27] jacket of racy white, hands enveloped in some strange wrapping. He slides the ring on the bride's finger while a bearded old man, dressed in oriental fashion, intones strange words, unknown to me, of which I hear quite a few *Eloim*!![28] The bride meanwhile remains in her wax doll state, immobile, with eyes closed. Next comes, if I'm not mistaken, the ritual of the glass cup filled to the brim. The rabbi [4-c] wets his lips and again sings something; an individual who assists him and looks to be a sacristan of the synagogue swallows a good half of the glass—they say that's not part of the ritual but it is so hot. Then comes the moment when the glass should be broken. But the one from which they have drunk is a beautiful brand new glass; the so-called sacristan more or less cleverly substitutes a chipped glass, which he hurls to the floor where it breaks with a crash. It is the moment, if I'm not mistaken, for the reading or rather the *chant* (everything is sung) of the contract. It's a large illuminated parchment on which everything is written in Hebrew. At each corner of the parchment, a hand is drawn, the palm side facing out; the two last fingers, side by side, are separated by a space of 2 or 3 centimeters from the first two also joined together—what does that signify? I've seen similar hands in metal hanging in the synagogues of the quarter. But the fingers were not separated that way.

[4-d] During all this time, the modulated moaning, which has had such an effect from the outset of the ceremony, resonates. The bride, always looking like a wax doll, left the room. I think they are taking her to get undressed in the room where

she was dressed and where the nuptial bed stands with its thick gauze curtains drawn. They set up a table where strange meats are served which we will have to taste shortly, for we are well and duly guests. When the members of the family finish, which won't be long, it will be our turn. We must do it—Our turn has come. We take a place at the table. They pour us a sort of *aguardiente*[29] which we taste just with our lips—hard-boiled eggs, cakes, pieces of preserved squash [*courge confit*] and other curious confections which we appreciate with mixed results. We leave most of it on the plate. But we have done our duty—yes, our duty as guests and sightseers [*curieux*] at 38 to 40 degrees.

[5-a] Meanwhile the bride has taken her place on the bed. She has changed her costume. She is in the middle of the bed her back to the wall squatting in oriental style. Now she has her eyes open. They are doubtless beautiful, but everything is obscure under the curtains. On her right and left, also squatting, are other women, the mother on the left. Each of us passes in front of the bed and extends our hand of congratulation, first to the mother, then to the daughter. Where has the groom gone? We do not see him any longer; it seems, for the moment, that he is no longer involved. The ceremony is not finished; there will be much more rejoicing. But time is going by and we have many more things to see. We must go dine more seriously and, above all, at any price, get out of this cauldron.

[5-b] So we leave. We cross the square again, and are soon back at the inn; we have lunch rapidly and off we go again.

Buison, Jean and Jeanne go off shopping. As for me, I take the opportunity to set up in front of the Spanish pharmacy sitting as comfortably as possible, under a veranda, where the free consultation customarily takes place. I'm seated there between the pharmacist, M. X, and the doctor M. X Barada,[30] both in the service of the Spanish ambassador. They are Spaniards of Moorish origins: their father and grandfather still wear the attire of well-to-do Moors, and are very friendly, in Spanish. The two children studied in Madrid. Are they Catholics or not?

From my vantage point, one can survey the entire square, which is illuminated by the blazing sun, without being too hot. (It has been, they say, one of the hottest days of the month.)

[5-c] As it is market day, the distribution of medications is carried out on a rather large scale. Only the Jews come to receive medications or consultations. It seems that the Arabs do not. (I knew nothing nor was I able to learn anything about their *Talebs*.[31]) I look especially at what is going on in the square, first the space, then its contents. Opposite is the open door of a mosque—still opposite but toward the right, is the palace, topped by a sort of square tower, covered with a roof of green tile, recalling what is seen at Granada. In the distance the town extends toward the Kasbah, whose walls attach it to the stronghold—finally the mountains form the background of the scene [*tableau*]. On the right, the door of the consulate, which differs from others only by its inscription. Jutting above the top edge of the wall, a dome with a cross on top appears. They have built this dome rather high so that it can be easily seen. It is the convent church of an order of Spanish fathers, I don't know which one, that we are going to see tomorrow. They have been living there since the war under the protection of the consul [5-d]. The portal of the Jewish quarter is in the next corner of the square formed by the side with the consulate and the side with the pharmacy. On the side of the square to my left, 3 or 4 streets enter, among which is one where I will go later and which leads directly to one of the town's caravan shelters [*caravanserails*[32]], the largest, I think. It forms one of the sides of the main square. Beside the pharmacy a fountain flows where a lot of people come to draw water and quench their thirst—Jews and Moors and also a number of Kabyles[33]

who come in from the countryside on market day and will disappear tomorrow.

What is seen within the square interests me more. The Orient is not surpassed by Europe. All the people are Jews of Africa or Muslims, engaged in selling chickens and donkeys, including miniature ones [*microscopiques*], which can be carried away in your arms. There are people from the town and from the surroundings. Some have come [6-a] on camels of which 8 or 10 can be seen—they take up space, a camel does—in the neighboring *caravanserail*. There are young Moors wearing the fez and Moors with turbans. The nomadic Arabs or those from the countryside look rather like brigands in their hooded robes [*burnous*]. The women cover themselves with large straw hats and the *burnous* with the traditional slit revealing only their eyes—a few, the ugly ones, let everything be seen. They have a sort of hump on their backs. It is surely a package which the *burnous* conceals. This is proved by the fact that the package sometimes turns out to be an infant. In these cases, a slit is made in the back of the *burnous* through which the head and chest of the baby pass. All are women of the common people, I think. I haven't seen a single "lady" [*dame*] promenading. But they told me that you could see some on the merchants' streets. All this activity proceeds in a cool manner [6-b] without much noise, and everywhere the guttural language resonates. A circle forms at a corner of the square; in the middle a man moves about and is speaking. In spite of having to cross the square in full sunlight, I approach, thinking that it will be some snake eater, perhaps something like that. But I lack the courage to wait until the end of the show. It's too hot. Besides I easily realized that our man wouldn't be doing anything but what we often see in our Paris squares: "Come on MM, be brave with your money, fork it over! do you think I'm going to show you this and that for 5 *sous*, for 10 *sous*?—for shame—etc.

etc." And his assistants, seated in oriental style in the circle
around the charlatan, add music with their guitars and tambourines to suggest generosity and curiosity to the public. It
will perhaps [6-c] go on for a long time yet. I prefer to beat
a retreat to my observation point where I'll find shade and a
glass of cool water. Jean, Jeanne, Buison, and Bayonna arrive
from the commercial streets of the town where they have seen
marvelous things; they are cooked. It's time to dine again. Let's
go. *Au revoir, MM* doctor and pharmacist. The latter shows us
a few good photographs which we buy.[34]

Lunch is nothing special. We are very cheerful and very
pleased with all we have seen. There is just one small blemish
that we don't dare admit. No news; impossible to receive or to
send any. I advised Augustine[35] in advance that this would last
4 days. It will certainly be more, even if it goes quickly. That
very evening, we were to have a very pleasant surprise. The
governor would inform us that, with the help of the military
telegraph of Algersiras, they had transmitted 2 dispatches from
Madame Charcot—good news. The Tetuan sky [6-d] looks
more beautiful to us, the air lighter, the heat less intense, and
everything more interesting. That is to say from our perspective. How right are those who say that everything is within us
. . . provided, all the same, that something from outside arrives,
of course!!

We prolong the meal, we chat, we receive merchants
who bring in the purchases or propose more of them. Then
the arrival of the Spanish consul who graciously agrees to
guide us through the streets of the town to see the houses of
2 Moors, rich, so they say, who await us at home. His 2 daughters accompany him, and they soon get acquainted with Jeanne.
It is settled that these young ladies will visit the women while
we, naturally, will not enter those private quarters, that's clear.
We plunge into the labyrinth; the advantage of these narrow

streets is palpable, in **[7-a]** this climate, in this season. One
has shade; it is almost cool. Often the street is covered by an
arcade, at other times by a trellis. In the open places, the sky
is seen; it is very clear everywhere, and, good Lord, we don't
complain about the shade. Sometimes at the end of a street, a
minaret appears. The one in the Kasbah on top of its rock is
most impressive. On the right and the left, we can't tear our
eyes away. Everywhere, the merchants look serious and, most
often, distinguished, even when they are shoemakers, black-
smiths, grocers, gunsmiths, etc. squatting in their little shops
swarming with objects for sale. They look at us absentmindedly,
probably mocking us. An old book dealer is engaged in reading a large book, perhaps the Koran. We put on **[7-b]** a show
of wanting to buy something from him; he doesn't even turn
his head and, continuing to read, he makes it understood by
a gesture that we are bothering him and he will sell nothing.
Here and there is a mosque with an open door. The entrance
is blocked by a plank, on which a bunch of street urchins
are leaning. But it is easy to glance down the peristyle where
the basin for ablutions sits, then into the sanctuary, always
constructed on the model of the cathedral of Cordova, on a
smaller scale, of course. I even managed to see the Mihrab[36]
several times in the rear! Lamps are hung (we have seen them
illuminated at night several times, in particular on the day of
our arrival) and alas, also, sometimes a few of those big brilliant silver balls with which the bourgeoisie in our country, who
lack taste, decorate **[7-c]** our gardens. We stop at times to look
with curiosity at all that. No one objects. However, sometimes
an old bigot, squatting in a corner, stares at us with a certain
threatening look which indicates clearly that, if we defied the
regulations, he would make it his business. Sometimes, not
far from the mosques, a door, always open, gives access to a
place where one finds a certain number of water closets, with

doors, and a hole level with the ground. A place is set aside for a pool in which the Arab goes up to wash his lower legs in the water. Water flows everywhere in those places, and it doesn't smell too badly.

Soon we arrive at one of our "wealthy Moors."

Suddenly there are no more shops. We wind our way down a corridor like so many we have seen [7-d], and, finally, come to a door in no way different from the others. I even notice that the street here is just as badly paved—kinds of stones with a sort of gutter in the middle as at Algeciras and Ceuta—they cut into your feet—and as poorly maintained as everywhere else. Mule and donkey droppings; and spider webs on the façade, and no one cares very much. That seems to me to be typical. Nothing distinguishes the door of the wealthy (doubtless for caution's sake). When walking around the streets, the only things which attract attention by way or ornamentation, except for the shops, are the doors of the mosques and, from time to time, the charming colored fountains which show to best effect at the crossroads.

But to come back to our visit: we knock, the door opens, and we are in an antechamber [8-a] which already exudes an atmosphere of comfortable living. The parquet floor along with the side walls to hand height are made of those tile mosaics recalling those of Granada. There are benches, also of mosaic, to the right and left. A 2nd door opens and we are in the patio, richly decorated in the same fashion. It is cool, it is charming, it's immaculately clean. Water flows continuously into a small basin in the center where limpid water stirs. The ground, like the walls up to hand height (columns above), is paved with those charming mosaics: one wouldn't dare walk on it in boots. Our hosts provide *babouches* [slippers]. A hole at the 4 corners of the patio permits the passage of the trunk of a beautiful orange tree which thrusts upward toward the *azotia*, there to find abundant daylight. The rooms are closed by those large double doors [8-b] that we already became acquainted with at the Spanish inn. A few are open. No decoration is visible. There are only mirrors, here and there, of every style, a veritable collection. Or, again, clocks of every type: there are cathedral clocks; many surely come from the Boulevard St. Denis.[37] They clash harshly with the native décor which is very fine, very delicate, the variety of which can be admired on the doors, large or small, where flowers and decorations of every kind are painted in the best taste. The walls above the tile are blank: but we are shown how, in the winter time, they are partially covered with bright colored fabrics whose placement recalls those draped fabrics [8-c] painted on the walls of our cathedrals restored according to the style of the period. Perhaps they really existed in the past, and not merely in painting.

The young ladies go into the women's quarters. Employing a searching gaze, we look into everything open to us. I think they were expecting us; most certainly, they were waiting for us. However a flurry of emotion, doubtless feigned, a pretended surprise, took place when we entered. A lady of mature years, who appeared beautiful to me, quickly fled, but not before showing us her face. That left 4 or 5 negresses, who shamelessly stayed where they were. Moreover, they were very beautiful, their arms and legs nude, their bodies lightly clothed in a clear fabric. They certainly do not belong to the religion whose acolytes cover up. As always, the first floor with balcony is just about the same as the lower floor. But it seems we cannot visit since the private living quarters are there. I look everywhere for a certain spot which interests me from a hygienic perspective. Instinct guides me. Here water flows on the ground—one certainly cannot go in without clogs. The floor is made of tile mosaics as are the walls—no seat—only a hole which seems narrow to me at ground level. One has to be agile—but the Arabs certainly are in this respect. They do everything squatting. It is perfect, a paradise for the senses of sight and smell.

Our host who has welcomed us graciously speaks Spanish. It is time to leave. The ladies return and try in vain to describe the marvels they have seen. We shake hands and head for the second wealthy Moor's house.

[9-a] We plunge once again into the labyrinth of streets and cannot get enough of looking everywhere. There is the neighborhood of shoemakers, of gunsmiths, cloth merchants, etc. At any rate, these classifications exist in principle. Painters on wood who produce beautiful chests [armoires] with interesting pictures are numerous. Their work is sometimes quite fine; the tones are brilliant—indeed, I would like to have those workers paint my doors and ceilings at Neuilly.[38]

Here we are at our 2nd Moor's. The door does not differ from what we have seen earlier. We enter: same antechamber. The arrangement of the patio is a little different. Again the patio has columns, tile, and the central basin. But, up high, there is a striking sort of cupola whose ornamentation in the form of stalactites recalls the Alhambra. They tell me that the owner is a [9-b] modernist and that his house is in the modern style. The decoration however [illegible word] strange borrowings. As the patio is not open to the sky, it follows that they do not have trees there. On the other hand, the fortunate arrangement of numerous windows, open wide and nearly touching one another, throws open entirely one side of the patio. This permits a view of the garden in the foreground, then the countryside stretching away as far as the eye can see. The house is located near the ramparts on the side where we will be departing the day after tomorrow. One can make out the plain where the Rio Martin flows, the square white customs house at a distance of 2 or 3 leagues perhaps, Martin's tower where we will embark, God willing, and, finally, the sea which will carry us to Ceuta.

I carefully inspect the little garden on which the bay windows I just mentioned open. It is extremely well cared for. The raised paths are paved with mosaic tiles in blue, white, mauve, and green, as elsewhere. Between the alleys where the earth appears always well watered, there are orange trees, pomegranates, etc., no palm trees. Types of wood structures in the form of trellises, support jasmine, which would not be able to stand on its own. A veritable boudoir of a garden, very amusing.

A kind of room or gallery separates the windows from the patio. I see 2 beautiful brass beds there, probably from England. It doesn't look like anyone sleeps there. Perhaps they are curiosity pieces. They must sleep on the soft cushions forming a divan that we see in all the other rooms. Here the collection of mirrors and clocks is most abundant. It's dreadful. But we ourselves collect the knick-knacks of others; why shouldn't they collect ours? I wouldn't be surprised to see a flowered chamber pot on a shelf [9-d]. Same ceremony for the ladies—same courteous farewells, and we are going back home delighted with what we have seen.

Here we are back at the inn; we dine heartily—no Arab meats, no *kouskousou*,[39] but good Spanish food. It was arranged that we would go to the Moorish café in the evening to hear music. We set out through streets as black as pitch. Tach Tach precedes us with his lantern. We meet a few strollers here and there, also with lanterns. Not many. Everybody is at home. We hear singing here and there accompanied by guitar and tambourine. Here we are in front of the café: I don't know what's wrong; he [the café proprietor] is in a bad mood. He has no one at his place, closes the shutters and slams the door in our face [*à notre nez et barbe*]. We wind up seated on a bench trying to figure out how we can best spend the evening. At this point, one of those shouting wandering *fools* [*ces fous errants*], several [10-a] of whom we met at the market this morning, goes by.

This one is quiet, he mutters something incomprehensible to me. We give him a few *sous*; he says thank you, probably, and disappears under the obscurity of an archway. Meanwhile we agree to send for tea from another place and to have the musicians come to the inn. Once again we will have the aromatic tea with which we became familiar at the Moroccan border, this time with green herbs floating in it. We head back to the inn. The musicians, numbering 4, accompany us. They set up in the patio. There is a violinist, he's the leader; they tell me he's the Tetuan corporal. He plays his instrument the way the bass is played, with great skill. There is a guitar player: a large flat mandolin which he only tunes in the morning and evening, its thick cords producing raucous tones. There is [10-b] a "Basque drum?" Finally, a kind of drum, shaped like a top, on which one taps with the palm side of the fingers. I think I saw one at Ceuta. Now they are squatting and looking serious. The leader wears a *burnous* and a white turban, as does the guitar player. The others wear the *fez*. They tune up as a prelude; then comes the chant. They seem to encourage each other: finally, they begin. They appear to know well what they are doing. There is a couplet, 2 couplets; they go on forever. Each couplet ends abruptly when one least expects. I try to understand, the harmony of course, not the words. I don't really follow. I prefer the Sevillans. They play another piece. It is pretty much the same thing . . . I feel a little tired and, without saying a word to the group, [10-c] stealthily, I go up to bed, delighted with my day.

12th August—5th day. [fig. 7]
3rd day at Tetuan: As usual, it is a beautiful day when the light enters through the crack in my door. This morning we are going to visit the house of a wealthy Jew in the Jewish quarter and the school and whatever else is interesting.

The Jew's house—who by the way is an old rascal [*filou*]—is basically similar to the Moor's. Same general structure, patio with columns, an upper floor, but it is less opulent and dirtier. No tiles on the floor, nor the walls. We are offered an alcoholic beverage and pastries, neither of which do I recognize. He is trying to soften us up for buying. We do not let ourselves be had. One of the girls puts on a costume like we saw yesterday at the wedding to show to Jeanne [10-d]. They pilfer some professional services [*consultations*] from me. These people are all eczematous, arthritic, puffy, scrofulous. Two infants a few months old have indurated and inflamed swellings in their groins. They look to me to be complications from circumcision.

The old Jew sought to offer us a pittance for these multiple examinations. He doesn't want to part with anything. I retaliate by writing down—*no charge*—he couldn't care less.

We go on to the school where they teach French and Spanish. It is a Jewish school supported by an international society in which French people certainly predominate.[40] The teachers have been students in France. I try to get them to say something to show that they retain an emotional bond with the country where they lived and whose language they teach: *nothing*, they are *heimatlosen*,[41] no homeland, at home everywhere. There are boys and girls [11-a]. The Moors never come to these schools, although nothing prevents them. So, I said that I wanted to see an Arab school. Impossible; the school was not open, it was the holiday.[42] From the Jewish quarter we go pay our visits to the Spanish consulate, and we take the opportunity to visit the Turks who show us their church and their Arabic library. After a few turns about the streets, we return home for lunch.

It is agreed that I will give a few medical consultations: they implored me to do so. A few people have been referred by the consul, or by M. Alvans, the military envoy, who never tires of being helpful, or by Bajonna.

Here come the patients, 5 or 6 of them, all Jews. They file into the patio. I sketch one who [11-b] presents a beautiful case of Parkinson's [**figs. 13 and 14**]. Nothing very interesting from the point of view of diagnosis. But all are nervous cases [*des nerveux*]. Yesterday, on the square, they showed me a Jew who remained mute, so they say, during his entire childhood but who eventually began to speak. Was he a case of hysteria?

The consultation is over. I must see the town some more so as to take with me an indelible visual impression. Along the way, on one of the most densely inhabited streets, we hear in the distance a sort of chanting, mixed and monotonous at the same time: the voices of men. They appear in a cortege of about a hundred persons; they are walking quickly, they seem to be in a hurry. "The dead go quickly" [*Les morts vont vite*].[43] In fact it is a burial. The deceased is carried on a kind of cot, nude in a white shroud which hides him completely, the head too. It seems to me that no one stirs nor extends greetings. We don't [11-c] either: that is not the custom here. We let the cortege pass, we will meet it again momentarily, at the cemetery.

We agreed that at 4 or 5 o'clock we would take up the invitation of a wealthy Moor, a client of Dr. X, whom we had already visited yesterday in his town house. He was waiting for us in his country house located perhaps a kilometer away from the town. It was interesting to go into one of those bamboo enclosures, which looked impenetrable, many of which we noticed the evening of our arrival in Tetuan. And then, after seeing how life goes on in town, it was good to see what country life might be like. We left by the gate [blank in text] the one which they had formerly shut in our face. It is not the shortest path to the country house, but we will have the benefit of going right along the low walls of the cemetery. We will see from afar—since the holy place is off limits to Christian dogs—the burial of the fine fellow whom we had just seen go by. It is also an opportunity to see the old cemetery [11-d] again in broad daylight and more peacefully. It consists of tiers of gravestones outside the walls along the hill topped by the Kasbah. Several tombs are impressive by reason of their size and style. The largest are on the summit of the hill where they stand out against the sky. Here and there are people apparently praying. They say that these are the tombs of the original Moorish leaders who, when banished from Granada, took refuge in Tetuan. The modern cemetery is on the other side of the road. One looks in vain for monuments like those seen in Turkish cemeteries at Constantinople. Here, for the poorest, there are simply stones placed side by side to form an oval around the earth where the dead person is buried. For others a low whitewashed wall, a sort of enclosure, surrounds a small garden with a few bushes piously cultivated. Nothing monumental, merely poor, but clearly with excellent intentions. We see everything without difficulty. The wall around the field where we are not allowed to enter is barely 2 meters high. In the [12-a] distance we see the burial of our man. Always, the chanting: a few wreaths. It seems that, one by one, each person comes forward to place something, surely a bit of earth, on the grave. Soon it is done. They disperse, one after the other, and, before long no one is left. It's all over quickly. Yet piety is displayed for the dead. I see women hovering around the grave that I just described. But we must get to our Moor's. It's 8 or 10 minutes further along the walls of the town. We follow a path bordered on the right and left by walls of bamboo similar to those we have already seen many times. Finally we are shown a door which Tach Tach recognizes and it is open. A wooden door framed in masonry. The garden is rather poorly tended: there are orange trees, pomegranate trees, supports for jasmine. The trees are raised above ground level [12-b] along rows to which water is conducted to keep them moist. We arrive at the house where they are waiting for us. A square house, whitewash paint, with an *azotia*, as usual; a single floor above the ground floor. In front, a terrace paved with the familiar mosaics; a bench, also covered with sections of tiles, is around the terrace. All this very pretty, very comfortable, and very easy to clean—but that is neglected. From this terrace, which is not raised more than 2 meters above the ground, one commands a view of the whole extent of the garden. Near the house is a well. This house, which we enter later, is extremely well cared for inside. It is adorned with mosaics like the wealthy houses visited yesterday. But no furniture here. These gentlemen do not live here. They are satisfied, no doubt, with coming to avail themselves of the open air from time to time, during the hot season [12-c]. But a Jewish servant seems to live here. She is the one who prepares everything necessary for the tea we are going to be served momentarily. Our host and his friend are seated near us. The older one prepares himself the aromatic tea with which we are already acquainted; he stuffs some leaves of a fresh plant, unknown to us, in the tea pot. We drink this tea with pleasure; 3 cups and cakes to go with them. The younger of our hosts is a tall man, slender, highly distinguished bearing, very elegantly attired: he speaks Spanish well. He slips away, discreetly gathers a few flowers in the garden and makes a bouquet which he offers to Jeanne, very gallantly and very discreetly. He resembles my friend, Mohammed Beinam. I would very much like to talk with him. But he does not know French and, as for me, I don't know Spanish[44] . . . nor Arabic. In a corner we see the illustrious Tach Tach, taking advantage of a favorable moment, to help himself without an invitation to 3 or 4 cups of tea, one after the other. But I think he gets on well with the Jewess.

Before leaving this very pleasant place we go up on the
azotia to see the landscape and especially to witness the sunset
behind the Kasbah. We see the old cemetery, which somehow,
why I don't know, always attracts the eye, fall into the shadows
bit by bit. I glance over to the Jewish cemetery, not far away,
where the mass of white tombstones creates an effect of white
laundry drying in the open air.

We return to town on foot with our hosts. We enter by
the large gate, the main one, on the side where more modern
fortifications seem ancient, bleached and readied. A badly
paved and bumpy road leads there. We follow a winding street
where there are no shops—an ornamental polychromatic
fountain appears opposite the gate. A little further on, I notice
an open window, but **[13-a]** closed by a wooden grill where a
bunch of small scapularies are hanging similar to those in our
Christian reliquaries. It is a small sanctuary where a lamp pro-
viding cloudy illumination is burning. On the right is another
winding street, also without shops. This definitely is not a commercial quarter. At this street, after shaking hands, our hosts
go off. Meanwhile, night has fallen. It happens rapidly here.
We come to the main square, and we return to the inn where
dinner awaits.

Today, once again, we have not wasted our time and we
are getting better acquainted with Tetuan, which we must leave
tomorrow.

After dinner, a number of farewell visits. One is of exceptional importance. All of a sudden, the most beautiful lantern
of colored glass that we have yet seen appears, followed by the
Moor of the consulate. He advances slowly with an imposing
bearing, a **[13-b]** cane in the hand not carrying the majestic
lantern. He pompously announces the Spanish consul who
soon appears, followed by his two daughters. I don't know why
this parade of lanterns reminds me of the 2nd act of *Oberon*[45]

and the charming marching music, chorus and accompaniments marking the steps of the patrol.

Farewells are prepared; some are deferred until tomorrow morning!

However, a few raindrops fall in the patio. The weather is changing. Will the wind be favorable for us to depart by sea or will we again have to trek by mule 12 or 14 hours!! Bajonna claims that the forecast is favorable. The skiff has arrived from Ceuta. It awaits us down there, near Fort Martin. Shall we go from there? That we will know tomorrow. We can't do anything about it [13-c]. So let's go to bed and sleep soundly.

13 August Next morning around 6 ½. I open my eyes and I see the sun. I get up and am soon ready. I go up on the *azotia* where there is a magnificent view. It's windy—is it a favorable wind?

I do a sketch [**fig. 16**] of what one sees of the town on the side of the Kasbah—the castle, the large mosque and its minaret, then a group of small mosques. This morning, all are flying a red flag, which floats in the wind. Today is a holiday; it's Friday.[46] All night long, they have been decorating, and very early, I heard a cannon fire. One also hears little concerts on the doorsteps of the mosques. We will see all this shortly.

From here, the square tower of the castle, covered with green bricks, shows to good effect. Yesterday we visited the interior, half in ruins, but there are some beautiful remnants. Mold everywhere; fountains filled with ferns and centipedes [13-d]. Some kind of artisan occupies the patio; yesterday when we entered, the governor, surrounded by a certain number of his agents, was squatting under the door. They appeared to be counting money in broad daylight or something like that. At the same time, in the back of the courtyard, I perceived one of the faithful, on his knees, making strange gesticulations, in agitated prayer.

All that returns to mind as I do my sketch. I turn to the other side—to see the square and the Jewish quarter. I would relish doing another sketch for I am in fine form [*en verve*]. But time is pressing and lunch is served.

Meanwhile, on the main square, the mules are being readied. Some will carry provisions, the others will carry us. Our Tetuan friends wait for us there; a few will accompany us to the boat—farewell, *au revoir*—the cavalcade sets out—we leave the town on the side reduced to ruins by the bombardment, which we visited yesterday [14-a]. Hovels everywhere, crumbling. It's gloomy and sad; destroyed nearly 20 years ago, and nothing rebuilt since. We come to a portal, cross it, and from there follow an old wall looking quite picturesque. We come to the plain which leads to the sea. Tetuan from here strikes us as picturesque; I keep turning around to see it again. As it recedes and recedes, I take it in better and better. We approach the country house where we were yesterday. At a turn in the path, Tach Tach appears, come to say his farewell. As we proceed, the land becomes more and more arid—at times a sandy desert. However the Rio Martin is a rather big river. We arrive at the customs house—we left at 10 o'clock and it is nearly 1 o'clock and we still have ½ hour on the path to reach [14-b] Tower Martin where Bajonna's skiff awaits. A crew of four men comes on board. The wind is good—our 2 Moors of the King are returning to Ceuta with us. The wind is favorable. Soon it fills the sail—and we set forth. Time for lunch.

But once again I cast my gaze on Tetuan which has been so hospitable to us. I see it still outlined in white against the black background of the mountains; there is the high minaret, here the grotto of [blank in text], the Kasbah perched on its hill and the old cemetery alongside. Farewell, daughter of Granada; we shall soon pay a pious visit to your mother.

Let's get back to practical matters. So far the wind is good. If that keeps up, we could reach Ceuta in 3 or 4 hours. But will it keep up? Who knows! One must always reckon with the treacherous elements . . . false lethe water.[47] But hunger calls and, while the boat glides gently, we empty out the bags of provisions: there are plates, dishes, napkins, forks, nothing lacking: **[14-c]** Madame Juanna, whom I cannot praise enough, as much for her striking beauty as for her amiability, has taken good care of us. There is salt. The wine is good. But, while we eat, we keep moving further away. Tetuan is no longer visible, nor Tower Martin. We have come under an overhanging huge wall of peaked rocks. Should we stop in a cleft in the rocks? We will have calm water and be more comfortable for lunch. Although the sea is calm, the surface of the boat is shaky when it's moving. So we huddle up against the side, like Barbary pirates of olden times, ready to strike a nasty blow. The rock is somber, the water under the boat is so clear and transparent that enormous depths can be seen. Here and there, a few auks? With long beaks they pursue their hunting business. A big fish with red and yellow spines rises to the surface where it floats. It is sick or wounded; we haul it in. It is time to leave. Everyone is satisfied **[14-d]**. The wind blows strongly: water strikes against the boat and comes back at us in a heavy rain. We wrap ourselves up and huddle together. We shall arrive somewhat wet, but it doesn't matter, all is well. But then the wind falls off. Rowing becomes necessary. We definitely will not get there in 3 hours. In fact, by the time we approach the fishery, it is already night. But the lights of Bajonna's house are in sight: a quarter of an hour later, we are helped out of the boat—farewell, till tomorrow—and we take the path to the inn. After dining, we go to bed.

14 August—The following morning, we must be ready early. The boat from Ceuta leaves at 7 o'clock. We go down the main street leading to the port—once again, we see the Moors and the Jews who constitute perhaps a good third of the population of Ceuta.

Bajonna accompanies us to [15-a] the boat. Aaron the Jew departs with a melancholy look. Did the tip strike him as inadequate? However, it was decent. He will get over it.

Farewell. The boat leaves. We will be in Algeciras in 3 hours. The sea is as calm as Baptiste[48] in the strait. I look at Ceuta fade away in the distance. The jetty, the town on the peninsula that links it to Morocco. In Ceuta there are 3 or 4 palm trees. Not a single one in Tetuan or its surroundings. I see once more old Ceuta, the fortified barracks, the Spanish towers perched on the frontier peaks—in back, the somber valley separating Spanish territory from Morocco—*adieu* or *au revoir* . . . who knows?

Time passes: now we turn our eyes toward the European coast. There's Gibraltar, there's Algeciras. Bit by bit the town comes into view. Here's the port where Burty [15-b] is that little black dot over there on the jetty—it gets bigger, bigger, fatter and soon attains its normal volume which, as you know, is not slight. It is he himself . . . there, sadly, all alone . . . yes, all alone . . . his bad angel has cowardly deserted him after having done his deed.

So, our poor friend, as a result of a deplorable suggestion by a hypochondriac of a consul, was stuck cooling his heels for a week in a sorry provincial town, while the rest of us return filled with charming and unforgettable memories. That is what happens, my friend, when you let yourself be frightened off by gossip of the port . . . yes, I remember, when we left, the wind was coming *from the east*, Gibraltar had *its cap*, the sea was a bit rough . . . but all things considered, our little African trip

[15-c] was well worth 2 hours of sea sickness which, perhaps, would not have occurred. And when you go to England, you aren't so fastidious.

Thus you have no excuse and are a bit pale and disheveled. You look wretched despite the beautiful blue cravat with white dots that you bought to make an impression in the bawdy houses of Algeciras. Oh, you poet, you!! What a lesson!! And how will you get out of it, when they ask you for news of Africa? For you cannot plead illness to physicians. Your only recourse is to face the sarcastic comments. O Scipio the African,[49] Oh count of Algeciras and Tetuan!!!!. This is what happens when you let yourself be terrified by *Gibraltar's cap*!

Tomorrow we will set out from Gibraltar for Malaga. And from Malaga we will go to Granada to pay the promised visit to the mother [15-d]. Visiting Granada after Tetuan is indeed logical. They say that many Tetuan people keep the key to their houses in Granada, hoping to return one day. When the Moroccan ambassador visited Spain, they tell me, he remained unmoved by Cordoba and Toledo; but in Granada, in the Alhambra, he was overwhelmed by feelings he could not hide. He requested the others to step aside for a moment, and he began to weep copiously!!!! Those present cried too.

Tetuan is Granada and Granada is Tetuan. As well, Granada is still a Moorish city; the nonchalance of its people, their love for letting things sort themselves out, all that recalls the Moorish rule. This is true to such an extent that when one has seen Tetuan and, from the heights of the Generalife,[50] one looks at Granada, it is not difficult, with a little imagination [*un petit effort de vision interne*] to reconstruct the Granada of the 15th century.

NOTES

1. Spanish: pier.

2. Possibly Jules Arène, brother of Paul, who served in the diplomatic corps as vice consul at Sousse in Tunisia. See Introduction, note 31, and Paul Arène, *Vingt Jours en Tunisie*, (Paris: Lemerre, 1884).

3. See Introduction, notes 20 and 31.

4. A physician and sometime traveling companion of the Charcots.

5. Jaime Bajonna or Bayona of Ceuta, the son of the fishing entrepreneur, served as guide to the Charcot party. Jeanne Charcot wrote to her mother: "M. Bayona is very nice and very helpful to us, he speaks a little Arabic and knows the countryside, the lodgings and Tetuan like the palm of his hand. Without him we would certainly got stuck en route." [*"M. Bayona est très gentil et il nous est très-utile, il parle un peu arabe et connait le pays, l'hôteliere et Tetuan comme sa poche, sans lui nous serions certainement restés en route."*] Subsequently, Jaime Bayona wrote to Jeanne Charcot with further information on Tetuan. He hoped to visit Paris soon and asked the young woman if she would send to him "the work that he has written on nervous diseases. I would be delighted to have it" [*"l'ouvrage qu'il [Charcot] a écrit des maladies nerveuses. j'aurais vrai plaisir de le posseder."*] (Undated letter in Charcot-family papers).

6. Guy de Maupassant, *Au Soleil*, in *Œuvres Complètes Illustrées*, vol. 9, (Paris: Librairie de France, 1934), p. 4, also decided to visit Algeria at the height of summer in 1881 for journalistic motives. Charcot's choice of season was determined by his son's need to be back in Paris for his medical studies well before the father's academic duties began in the autumn. Apparently they experienced some of the hottest days of that summer in Morocco with their estimates of temperatures ranging from 40 degrees centigrade (Charcot), and 45 (Jean-Baptiste), to "50 et plus qu'il fait au soleil" (Jeanne, who seemed to suffer most).

7. *La Gran Via* composed in 1886 by Federico Chueca of Madrid. Jeanne Charcot wrote to her mother: "During the two nights spent at Ceuta only papa et Buison were able to sleep and yet not more than one or two hours, thanks to the heat, the mosquitoes,

the fleas and the flies [*depuis deux nuits que nous couchons à Ceuta il n'y a que papa et Buison qui ont pu dormir et encore pas plus d'une ou deux heures, grâce à la chaleur, aux moustiques, aux puces et aux mouches*].

8. Question mark in text.

9. Emphasis in original.

10. Italian: abandon all your hope. The famous line comes from Dante's *Inferno*, canto III, line 9.

11. Italian: of the first rank. Emphasis in original.

12. Charcot's colorful phrase about these innocent looking inmates literally translates as "to whom one would give the good Lord without confession" [*auxquels on donnerait le bon Dieu sans confession*].

13. caravan

14. This was evidently a most embarrassing role reversal for the neurologist, accustomed to looking at female patients in a state of undress.

15. Paris street in the 10th arrondissement known for its shops selling crystal ware, porcelains, and china. As a keen collector, Charcot would have been quite familiar with such items of domestic French production.

16. See Introduction, note 68. Jeanne wrote that her brother, the future explorer, at the time a beginning medical student, was perhaps the least eager of the group to return: "He's beginning truly to love traveling, and then going home means for him one exam after another" [*il commence à véritablement aimer voyager, et puis le retour pour lui veut dire concours sur concours*].

17. Jeanne's letter of Wednesday, August 11, described their caravan from Ceuta to Tetuan the previous day from her own perspective with slightly different details: "We left on five mules, eight other mules carried the bags, tents, provisions, two Moors belonging to the Spanish army in full regalia, two other Moroccan Arabs armed, and a Negro of the most beautiful blackness constituted our escort, plus three mule drivers [*Nous sommes partis sur cinq mulets huit autres mulets portaient les sacs les tentes et les provisions, deux Maures appartenant à l'armée espagnole en grand costume, deux*

autres Arabes du Maroc armés, et un nègre du plus beau noir formaient
notre escorte, de plus trois muletiers].

18. Don Juan Prim (1814–70), Spanish general, one of the leaders of
the expedition that captured Tetuan in 1860.

19. Probably an allusion to the Biblical miracle of the Israelites crossing the Red Sea on dry land.

20. Charcot did retain the newspaper for his album where it can
still be seen at Neuilly. Despite the amusing bathos in this passage: "what a come-down," from pleasant reveries on the virgin
spring of Lucretius upon seeing the soiled newspaper, Charcot's
contempt for the most widely circulated Paris daily was genuine.
The columnist, Ignotus of *Le Figaro*, had published a biting
satirical lead article against the neurologist in 1883, protesting
Charcot's nomination to the Academy of Sciences.

21. Another instance of Charcot's extreme affection for animals,
a sentiment that in part accounted for his dislike of animal
experimentation.

22. For a similar experience at the gates of Tetuan, fifty years earlier, see Charles Didier, "Le Maroc," *Revue des deux mondes* 8
(november 1836), 250.

23. Charcot omits *closing* quotation marks to his speculative interpretation beginning with "Christian dogs..." of what has been
shouted, probably in Arabic incomprehensible to him.

24. Spanish: a terrace or platform on the flat roof of a house.

25. Jeanne Charcot described Madame Juanna as "*une juive espagnole.*"
Thus her father here was evidently mistaken in his belief that he
could readily identify Jews. It appears that Pierre Loti stayed in
the same inn a short time later. He refers to an "*auberge espagnole*"
recommended by his guide: "I expected some filthy hole, instead
it turned out to be a large Moorish house white washed and imma-
culate. The hostess, as beautiful as a statue, under her Jewish
coiffure, welcomed me with a smile . . ." [*j'attendais quelque bouge*
malpropre et immonde: au contraire c'est une grande maison mauresque
toute blanche de chaux imaculée. Une hotesse, belle comme une statue,
sous sa coiffure juive, m'accueille avec un sourire . . .]. *Cette éternelle*
nostalgie. Journal intime, 267.

26. Jews who held consular positions wore European clothes in order to circumvent the Muslim restrictions forbidding them to wear anything but black. See Didier, 254.

27. The *tallit* or Jewish prayer shawl.

28. Hebrew: The Lord.

29. Spanish: generic name meaning "firewater" or literally "burning water" of clear drinks between 29% and 60% alcoholic content.

30. Presumably brothers. Julio Barrada, a Tetuan physician, was the son of a naturalized Spanish consular agent and a Spanish woman. See Miège, 304–5, n. 9.

31. Arabic for learned persons who worked as scribes and presumably healers. The term also referred to the first level university degree.

32. Term derived from Turkish, literally "caravan palace."

33. A Berber people whose traditional homeland was in northeast Algeria.

34. Six photographs of Tetuan are in Charcot's album of the trip at Neuilly. Their subjects include a street in the Jewish quarter and the house of a wealthy Moor. It is noteworthy that Charcot, an advocate of photography at the Salpêtrière, did not use the camera himself but, evidently, preferred to retain his visual impressions with sketches.

35. Madame Charcot's maiden name was Augustine Richard.

36. Niche in the wall of a mosque, which faces toward Mecca to indicate the direction for prayer.

37. Here again, a Parisian commercial street in the 10th arrondissement.

38. Charcot's summer house in the Paris suburb of Neuilly. See Introduction, 15 and note 42.

39. Didier, 253 described the local *kouskousou*: [*C'est le plat favori des Maures, une espèce d'étuvée composée de pates fines* (puntitas), *d'œufs durs, de poulet, d'agneau, de mouton, melés et bouillis ensemble. On saupoudre cela de safran, de poivre et autres épices fortes, et l'on sert le tout dans une immense patère à pieds*. . .].

40. The Alliance Israélite Universelle founded its first school in Morocco at Tetuan in 1862. See Norman A. Stillman, *The Jews of Arab Lands: a history and source book*, (Philadelphia: Jewish Publication Society of America, 1979), 308–9.

41. German: homeless. Charcot wrote the same word in the margin of his copy of Henry Meige's inaugural medical thesis on "*le juif errant*." See Introduction, note 79 In contrast to Charcot's opinion, Jean-Louis Miège, 331, wrote that the Alliance Israélite Universelle schools produced a generation of Jews imbued with "the principles of militant Western culture" [*les principes de la civilisation occidentale qui lutte*] who gained key places in Moroccan economic, administrative, and journalistic life.

42. Friday, the Muslim holy day.

43. The title of the book by Alexandre Dumas (Paris: Michel Lévy, 1861), a collection of eulogies.

44. This appears to contradict several other places in the journal where Charcot implies that he is able to communicate in Spanish. See B, 5-c and 9-a; A, 5-b. Probably he could understand and speak a little.

45. *Oberon, or the Elf King's Oath* (1826) an opera by Carl Maria von Weber. Act 2 opens in the splendid court of Haroun al Rachid with a chorus of praise to the Arab ruler. The opera remained popular throughout western Europe until the 1860s. A lavish production was mounted at Paris in 1857.

46. August 13 was in fact a Saturday.

47. English in text. Possibly another allusion to Dante's *Inferno* and the river of Lethe in the Underworld, which betrays memory.

48. *Tranquille comme Baptiste:* French expression signifying "exceptionally calm" originating in early nineteenth century most likely in reference to a stock figure named Baptiste or Gilles who maintained his calm in the face of violence or tumult.

49. Scipio Africanus, Roman general renown for defeating Hannibal of Carthage as well as for his fondness for beautiful women.

50. 14th century summer palace and estate of Muslim rulers in Granada.

III

French Transcription

Huit jours au Maroc. Ceuta et Tetuan

[Ms A][1-a] 1er jour. D'Algesiras à Ceuta

8 août 1887 – Vers midi après avoir bien déjeuné à la fonda des Quatro Naciones, où nous hébergeons depuis depuis 2 jours, pour quelque argent, M. Royi ancien maître d'hôtel de la Marine, nous descendons la grande rue d'Algesiras, précédés par nos petits colis. On va s'embarquer sur la [lacune en texte]. Qui porte le courrier d'Algesiras à Ceuta. Il doit partir vers une heure, mais le sort veut qu'à 3 heures nous serons toujours en rade.

Hier soir il a fait du vent; Gibraltar a son chapeau de nuages, – c'est le vent d'est- mauvais temps surtout en mer : d'ailleurs en face de l'hôtel toute la nuit la mer n'a cessé de se briser avec fracas a l'extrêmité de la calle del muelle où se voit l'ogive d'une vieille porte de fortification – vous le voyez la mer est **[1-b]** un peu houleuse dans le golfe, que sera-ce dans le détroit. Je ne m'embarquerais pas en ce moment; j'attendrais de 3 à 7 jours. C'est le compte avant de me mettre en route. D'ailleurs qu'allez vous faire à Ceuta; auberges abominables : j'y ai été assez mal reçu;

j'y suis arrivé le soir, j'en suis parti le lendemain matin sans y rien voir. Et puis Tetuan...mais ce n'est pas très sûr..., ainsi s'exprimait hier notre jeune consul et pendant qu'il parlait, je voyais notre ami B[urty] pâlir ses traits se tiraient... Je pensai qu'il éprouvait quelque malaise! Oui, il souffrait mais c'était moralement. Les derniers mots du consul l'avaient retourné, et avant de me coucher Buison d'un air de diplomate me fait la communication suivante : J'ai la mission délicate de vous dire que B ne viendra pas avec nous demain. Comment, bah, pourquoi? Il m'a prié de vous supplier de ne pas insister...C'est bon, je n'insisterai pas... et voilà pourquoi le lendemain matin **[1-c]** nous descendîmes 4 seulement au lieu de 5 dans la barque qui devait nous mener au Correo, adieu Burty, adieu Arène...amusez vous bien tout au moins et écrivez tous les jours à ma femme.

Buisson s'était mis en 4. Nous avions des lettres pour le directeur de la prison de Ceuta, pour le gouverneur, pour toutes les autorités plus ou moins constituées; et le gouverneur d'Algesiras nous promettait lui-même de faire jouer si besoin était et si possible était de faire jouer le télégraphe militaire en notre faveur. Il nous rattachait ainsi gentiment à l'Europe par une Espérance.

Nous voilà embarqués, 2 heures d'attente : on attend le courrier? Pourquoi ce courrier est-il en retard de 2 heures... chose d'Espagne. Enfin nous voilà partis; un peu de houle, mais personne de nous ne songe à être incommodé, pas même Buisson qui le craignait. Pauvre Burty la chose serait faite, car nous voilà en vue de Ceuta...mais hélas! Le chapeau de Gibraltar devait nous jouer un mauvais tour.

[1-d] Il est 6 heures. Nous sommes en retard de plus de 2 heures. Les gens qui devaient nous attendre en barque se sont fatigués. Nous descendons dans la barque commune assez mal emmagasinée; inconsciemment je fronce légèrement le sourcil... entrée ratée me dis-je in petto... C'est une erreur. Tout est pour le mieux, car sur le port, à mesure que nous approchons nous apercevons une 10ᵉ de personnes qui visiblement nous attendent et parmi lesquelles se distinguent par sa taille et sa tenue le directeur de la prison : excellent homme, grand, maigre très prévenant, orné d'une cravate impossible et d'un gilet blanc interminable qui mettent bien en relief sa bonne figure de Don Quichotte. Il y a là aussi et enfin Bajonna qui devait être notre providence pour l'expédition de Tetuan. Nos petits colis sont débarqués. Ils sont au nombre de 7, et sont immédiatement saisis par autant d'hommes de mine assez sinistre qui paraissent dirigés par un 8ᵉ homme de même mine ; ce sont des galériens, apprenons-nous chemin : mais vous pouvez avoir toute confiance. C'est bien, marchons !

[2-a] En outre, se fait remarquer de nous un grand vieux juif avec la lévite orientale. Viens avec moi me dit-il : je suis le guide de la fonda Espagnole. Tu auras besoin de moi — le juif me ferait l'effet, je ne sais pourquoi, de devoir s'appeler Aaron...Justement c'est bien là son nom.

Notre arrivée fait événement dans la ville. Tout le monde nous regarde. Quels sont ces originaux qui viennent fréquenter ce pays a cette époque de l'année — Ils sont fous... Inglès, Inglès. Non pas Inglès, disons nous, mais Français. Et nous ne sommes pas si fous que vous croyez : on le verra bien par la suite.

Chemin faisant on rencontre une foule des juifs, et également une foule des maures de toute condition : paysans, bourgeois, marchands : des marocains noirs et blancs : plusieurs poussant des ânes chargés de toutes sortes de choses. Nous voilà déjà en pays marocain : oui pour un bon tiers peut-être.

[2-b] Nous voilà arrivés devant une maison d'assez [mauvaise (mot rayé)] médiocre apparence ; en face le grand poste où les soldats de ligne espagnole prennent l'air. C'est la fonda Espagnole ; là seulement on a trouvé à nous loger. À la guerre, comme à la guerre ; nous ne sommes pas ici pour nous amuser — bravez toutes les vermines de la création : cela fait partie du programme. D'ailleurs comment nous plaindre, pour occuper l'appartement majeur de

la maison, en promiscuité avec les propriétaires dont il faut traverser la chambre à coucher, occupée par 3 personnes, ainsi que la cuisine qui loge une servante, lorsque la nature parle en nous d'une certaine façon à la vérité quand on a franchi tout cela on est récompensé de ses peines, car on trouve enfin une installation en plein air fort pittoresque.

Détails que tout cela; nous dinons pas trop mal en somme et le soir nous recevons, a l'heure du café, nos nouveaux amis de Ceuta [**2-c**] qui viennent s'entendre avec nous pour organiser les parties de demain – Cependant il se fait tard et nous allons nous coucher... bientôt le sommeil vient malgré la chaleur atroce, la crainte vague des insectes, et le retentissement bruyant du piano de Mlle X qui en face nous gratifie de quelques uns des airs de la pièce à la mode a Madrid, la Gran via.

2e jour La pêchérie et Les frontières du Maroc – Le bagne.
9 *août* 1887 – De père en fils en remontant les siècles à perte de vue, les grands pêchéries de l'almadrade (?) à Ceuta, sont entre les mains des Bajonna. C'est là où Bajonna fils nous conduit ce matin. Nous sortons de Ceuta par la côte sud-est, et nous voilà au bord de la mer, sous le rempart; dans une espèce de hangar où sont pendus en quantité innombrable des poissons, surtout des poissons volants desséchés. C'est là le magasin placé sous la surveillance de Bajonna, [**2-d**] père, vieillard de 65 ans, tout ratatiné, ridé comme une vieille pomme mais assez vert, cependant, bien qu'il souffre de l'estomac. Mais c'est la pêche elle-même qu'il faut voir. Les grands filets sont installés à un kilomètre peut-être de la plage; on aperçoit là bas les barques qui les portent et les pêcheurs qui tout à l'heure vont les lever. C'est là que nous allons; la mer est un peu houleuse et l'un de nos compagnons qui fait souvent cette partie, *pour s'habituer* est bientôt malade...honneur au courage malheureux! Nous voilà près des grands filets : le cercle des bateaux se referme à un signal donné, en même temps que de chaque bateau

on tire la [?] ; le cercle se rétrécit rapidement, les pauvres bêtes par centaines, pour la plupart ce sont des poissons volants, grouillent avec bruit en se frappant les uns les autres, montrant tour à tour leur dos d'acier et leur ventre d'argent ; quelques uns parviennent en se redressant comme des ressorts à sauter par dessus bord... bonne chance – mais pour ce qui est des autres, plus d'espoir... Lasciate ogni speranza, le souffle de la vie de ces pauvres bêtes s'exhale avec effort.

[ms B] [3-a] Ce n'est partout que convulsions et agonie : tout cela souffre et meurt, c'est affreux ; mais c'est la loi : La nature est immorale et les gros mangent les petits ou inversement.

Nous retournons à terre et nous nous rendons du côté du môle pour visiter le bagne : Le Bagne est partout dans la ville, parce que la plupart des galériens parcourent la ville surveillés par des espèces de chiourmes qui ne distinguent des autres que par un brassard. Mais c'est dans la prison que tout le monde demeure, et c'est là qu'il faut aller chercher si l'on veut les voir, ceux qui ne sortent jamais et ceux qui par punition portent des chaînes. L'installation est telle qu'on se la peut figurer : des grands dortoirs misérables et fétides ; des cours affreuses.

[3-b] Les détenus parmi lesquels on nous signale plusieurs scélérats *di primo cartello*, auxquels on donnerait le bon Dieu sans confession, ont une veste grise et un pantalon idem en toile, rien de jaune, rien de vert comme dans nos bagnes d'autrefois. De cet examen nous avons bientôt assez = Il fait très chaud d'ailleurs. Nous avons soif et faim. Nous rentrons à l'hôtel par une longue rue étroite, où les constructions rappellent celles d'Algesiras, avec la petite fenêtre grillée du rez de chaussée – propice aux amants. Chemin faisant, nous croisons soit des maures, des juifs et des galériens – mais nous sommes déjà faits à ce triple contact.

La 2e partie de la journée sera bien employée ; il s'agit de faire [3-c] la partie dite du Seraï, bien connue à Ceuta. Tous nos amis nous accompagnerons à cheval, ou à mulet. Une voiture, celle du gouverneur, nous conduira Jeanne, moi et Buison jusqu'à une certaine distance ; après quoi il nous faudra monter à mulet ou à cheval pendant près d'une heure.

Il est 3 heures environ ; on a laissé passer la grande chaleur. Cependant il fait si chaud que j'oublie toute réserve. J'ai laissé de côté cravate et faux cols ; je porte une chemise non empesée, pas de gilet, pour tout partage mon petit veston de soie qui me sert souvent de robe de chambre. Ce laisser aller, nous paraît justifié par cette circonstance que Jeanne à part, il n'y a pas des femmes avec nous..... Mais hélas ! Il y en aura des *femmes*... tout à l'heure. [3-d] Nous voilà partis. Nous franchirons les 3 enceintes qui protègent Ceuta du côté du Maroc... fortifications du 17e pour le moins, bonnes au plus contre les marocains. Nous entrons dans la campagne.

Le sol s'élève progressivement à droite et à gauche la mer, car nous sommes dans une presqu'île étroite ; devant nous une série de monticules et au fond de vraies et hautes montagnes à l'air sombre. Sur la droite on me montre la vieille Ceuta (romaine ?) où l'on voit des murailles antiques et où l'on trouve des mosaïques – ça et là quelques maisons de campagne – à gauche une petite mosquée qui paraît bien soignée – des maures vont et viennent sur la route et se mêlent aux Espagnols – nous [? arrivons mot illisible], et sur la gauche nous [4-a] apercevons un grand édifice carré qui est à la fort et une caserne. C'est là que nous devons faire halte et quitter la voiture pour prendre les mulets – Mais avant de descendre je me retourne et j'aperçois un des plus beaux paysages qu'on puisse voir. La ville de Ceuta, enceinte de murs, et le môle qui la termine se détachent sur le fond de la mer bleue, comme s'il s'agissait d'un petit plan en relief et dans le lointain on aperçoit Gibraltar.

C'est le moment de descendre ; hélas, il y a des dames en robe de soie bleue, avec falbalas et de très beaux militaires qui viennent au devant de nous, courtoisement. Où me fourrer ? Si j'avais su... etc. Ma foi, tant pis ; je passerai peut-être inaperçu au milieu [4-b] de tous les beaux cavaliers qui m'accompagnent – mais on me présente comme un personnage!!!!! Je fais la meilleure contenance possible évitant de mon mieux le regard des Dames...

Il est temps de partir. Jeanne et moi on nous place sur une mule... On me hisse sur une espèce de cacolet où je m'installe comme un infirme...que je suis : On n'est pas trop mal là dessus et je ne suis pas fâché de l'expérience car demain c'est ce métier là qu'il faudra faire pendant 12 ou 14 heures. La promenade d'aujourd'hui, pour la partie mulet va durer 2 h 1/2 environ. Je multiplie ce chiffre par la pensée par 7. Et après méditation [4-c], je conclus : ce sera dur mais cela ira.

Après le poste caserne, la route cesse, ce n'est plus qu'un chemin de mules : nous montons, nous montons toujours. Nous passons autour d'une des tours espagnoles, rayées verticalement de rangs qu'on aperçoit de distance en distance de Ceuta, signalant la frontière marocaine; il y a là dedans des soldats qui ne doivent pas s'amuser beaucoup à la longue; car le site devient à la fois désert, imposant et plutôt triste. Les montagnes d'en face, qui sont le Maroc sont noires et sombres et c'est par là que nous allons. Le chien jaune en forme de lévrier qui nous accompagne, que je prenais pour un chien d'Afrique n'est cependant qu'un chien de chasse d'Espagne. Il fait lever par ci par là des perdrix. [4-d] à la grande joie de la plupart de nos compagnons qui hélas en sont encore philosophiquement et moralement à cet état où ce sport sanguinaire qu'on appelle la chasse est considéré comme une partie de plaisir. Comme je fais ces réflexions s'ouvrent devant nous la petite vallée sombre où coule devant nous le tout petit ruisseau qui sépare le Maroc de la possession espagnole. Il y a là dans le fond des lauriers roses tout fleuris; mais de l'autre côté en face une montagne d'un vert sombre où s'étagent de superbes chênes lièges au feuillage noir : c'est imposant et un peu triste. Tout en haut du [?] une petite maison blanche et cossue où l'on distingue de loin des créneaux. C'est là que nous allons.

Le ruisseau est franchi. Nous voilà en Maroc. Personne excepté nous, ni d'un côté ni de l'autre. [5-a] Légère émotion, tout instinctive car Il n'y a absolument rien à craindre. Hier nous avons rencontrés à Ceuta où il avait affaire le chef du poste où nous allons ; il a fait annoncer notre arrivée à son fils aîné qui le remplace en son absence, et qui nous attend prêt à nous rendre tous les honneurs dus à notre rang.

Nous gravissons la colline avec confiance par un sentier, en zig zag ; le petit fort blanc et carré grossit à mesure qu'on approche et l'on ne distingue toujours personne. Enfin voilà 2 êtres humains qui se détachent sur le fond blanc de la maison carrée. Ils n'ont pas fort bonne mine ; l'un d'eux porte un fusil. Ils sont vêtus d'un burnous de couleur gris sale. Nous [5-b] montons toujours – on met pied à terre nous voilà arrivés : quelques hommes s'emparent de nos mules et nous pénétrons dans l'enceinte à demi vitesse du pauvre fort – après avoir traversé une cour, on nous introduit dans une petite chambre où nous trouvons le fils du chef, jeune garçon de 18 ans environ à l'air distingué, coiffé d'un fez qui se lève pour nous accueillir, avec toute sorte de politesses en nous tendant la main gracieusement. Dans un coin se trouve son jeune frère âgé de 12 ans. Les autres personnages sont de soldats du poste : nous nous accroupissons sur des coussins autour d'un plateau où se trouvent des tasses à café qui me paraissent venir de la rue de Paradis. La théière est plus originale, et surtout la petite boîte laquée, rouge où [5-c] un serviteur prend le thé. Car il s'agit de prendre une tasse de thé et du gâteau. Que dis-je, une tasse de thé, c'est 3 tasses qu'il faudra prendre : plus si l'on veut – moins jamais ! C'est ainsi que le veut la politesse, nous nous exécutons d'autant mieux que par cette température accablante ce thé aromatisé que nous retrouverons à Tetuan nous paraît excellent...... J'en aurais bien pris une 4e mais il se fait tard : le jour baisse, il faut retourner à Ceuta. D'ailleurs la conversation languit bien que tout le monde là parle un peu espagnol. On se dit adieu cordialement on nous hisse sur nos mules et nous voilà partis par la route qui nous a vu venir. Le jour baisse rapidement et quand nous arrivons à Ceuta il fait nuit. Nous dînons de [5-d] bon cœur et nous allons dormir à poings fermés, le plus vite et le plus fortement possible, car demain il faudra se lever à 5 heures et la journée sera rude.

3ᵉ *journée*
De Ceuta à Tetuan
– La Maison du Maure
– La porte de Tetuan fermée
10 août 1887
Le premier plan avait été de se rendre à Ceuta par mer, et c'est Bajonna sur son bateau qui devait nous conduire. Mais le vent n'était pas favorable. On sait quand on part par ce temps-là... on ne sait pas quand on arrive : pourrons nous franchir la barre du rio Martin. Etc., etc., voilà.

[6-a] Les doutes qu'on émettait certes, ajoutait-on, il n'y a aucun danger à courir. Si on n'arrive pas on reviendra. Toutes ces considérations ne me paraissaient pas plaider en faveur du trajet par mer. Par ce chemin là si nous réussissions nous aurions cela est vrai, l'avantage de n'être à cheval que pendant deux ou 3 heures ; mais nous risquerions peut-être de perdre 1 ou 2 jours et nous n'avions pas, à cause de Jean, de temps à gaspiller.

Le plancher des vaches est plus sûr ; ce sera long, pénible peut-être mais enfin nous arriverons à coup sûr. C'est ce dernier parti qui fut pris et exécuté – Nous reviendrons par mer ; le vent pendant ce temps là nous deviendra favorable.

[6-b] Il est cinq heures du matin, les mules nous attendent dans la rue. 2 mules portent les bagages et les provisions...car il faut manger et se vêtir...même en Afrique. Buisson, Jeanne et Bajonna chacun une mule sur laquelle ils se tiennent à califour-chon. Jeanne et moi chacun une mule à cacolet où nous sommes assis, installés en manière d'infirmes.... C'est pour moi que je parle,

car Jeanne a les infirmités naturelles à son sexe. 2 conducteurs espagnols et 2 maures du roi sans armes nous accompagnent. L'un de ces derniers, nous l'avons reconnu chemin faisant est un brave homme et un philosophe. Il y aussi un grand nègre, tout jeune, à l'air un peu effaré, rasé à l'exception d'une touffe de cheveux qu'il [6-c] porte sur la tempe droite. On le dit un peu idiot et fils d'un grand personnage dogonimi. Nous voilà cheminant à travers des rues de la ville et nous sortons par la porte des champs, comme hier – mais au lieu de prendre sur la droite nous prenons sur la gauche, longeant la mer dont nous ne nous écartons jamais beaucoup pendant toute la durée de notre voyage. Il fait chaud, mais le ciel est légèrement couvert par places. Peut-être ne cuirons nous pas absolument. D'ailleurs tout le monde s'est mis à son aise et ma toilette d'aujourd'hui reproduit exactement celle d'hier. En voilà pour 4 heures ; après cela nous ferons une halte à la maison du maure.... C'est à peu près moitié chemin. Là nous trouverons de l'ombre et de l'eau. Nous ferons halte pour déjeuner [6-d] et un peu la sieste ; puis nous repartirons frais et dispos.... Voilà le programme.... On verra qu'il a du être modifié légèrement sur quelques points. À gauche la mer, à droite des montagnes qui s'étagent et qui s'avancent ou reculent de façon à resserrer ou à élargir la plaine, quelques petites rivières à traverser, voilà la disposition du terrain de Ceuta à Tetuan. Pas de route proprement dit d'ailleurs. Des sentiers à peine tracés ; pas d'arbres, des buissons plus ou moins touffus et plus ou moins élevés représentant parfois de petits bois en miniature. Des lauriers roses quand il y a un rio. Pas de villages c'est le désert. En sortant de Tetuan quelques champs de maïs. Dans le lointain à mi-côte, sur la montagne, quelques cabanes, des hommes qui tamisent le blé et c'est tout [7-a] ce que nous voyons d'humain pendant les 4 ou 5 premières heures ; c'est à peu près tout ce que nous verrons pendant les 5 ou 6 autres.

Bientôt nous atteignons le 1e poste marocain, maison carrée qui domine une haute colline. De là se détachent 2 maures de l'empereur qui doivent nous accompagner; L'un d'eux porte un fusil, l'autre porte une besace. Ces 2 dessus ne se mêlent pas vraiment au cortège, tantôt ils s'approchent tantôt ils disparaissent – pour reparaître quelque temps après à un repli de terrain....décidément ce sont des fantaisistes; ils ont d'ailleurs assez mauvaise mine avec leur burnous qu'on croirait qu'ils ont trempé dans la suie.

[7-b] Il y a peut-être 2 heures que nous marchons. À un moment donné la plaine s'élargit. Au milieu l'on voit un castillo ruiné et recouvert de lierre – non loin des pierres rassemblées de façon à circonscrire un ovale de terre. C'est une tombe, il y en a beaucoup comme cela. Sur quelques unes d'entre elles on voit planté un bâton au bout duquel est suspendue une loque rouge, d'un rouge douteux, laquelle a du être autrefois d'un beau rouge : c'est le tombeau d'un chef, plus ou moins canonisé et porté à l'état de saint. En ce lieu a eu lieu la bataille contre les marocains qui a décidé la marche sur Tetuan. Il y a plus de 20 ans de tout cela et le nom de Prim revient à l'esprit. Nous marchons, nous marchons toujours; je regarde [7-c] quelquefois ma montre. Bientôt nous allons arriver chez le maure sans doute! Il est l'heure on a faim et soif. Mais où est cette diable de maison du maure : on ne la voit pas. Il y a ici quelques arbres et des rochers. On a perdu de vue la mer. On marche ainsi anxieusement pendant près d'une heure : diable de maison égarée. On commence à tancer les maures de l'empereur qui nous ont conduit par ce mauvais chemin. Enfin là voilà, c'est une hutte à peine élevée au dessus de terre, perdue, parmi les broussailles, les grands cactus et dont le toit ne la distinguait pas ni par la couleur ni par la forme des quelques rochers qui gisent çà et là. Le maure en ouvre la porte. C'est un homme de 60 ans à l'air assez distingué [7-d] mais misérable dans son [?]. Il est là avec une adorable petite fille de 5 ou 6 ans, qui fait la boudeuse et nous regarde cependant bien attentivement avec de petits yeux noirs comme le geai. C'est sa fille. Il y a un roman dans cette affaire : la mère et le père sont mal ensemble le 1e est à Tetuan; lui, le vieillard il aime

mieux la solitude que le séjour à la ville avec sa femme. Peu nous importe du reste = on dit que c'est un homme non sans fortune. Il serait issu d'une famille de Grenade et porterait avec lui « les papiers » qui le constituent propriétaire d'une maison de Grenade. etc., etc., quoiqu'il en soit il vit là dans une vraie hutte ; entourée d'un petit jardin fruitier. Il y a des poules.

[**8-a**] Dans la cour un grand figuier qui donne un peu d'ombre, dont on augmente l'épaisseur en tendant une toile : c'est là que nous nous installons pour déjeuner. Et l'on nous apporte de l'eau fraîche. Le programme est donc rempli au pied de la lettre : nous avons eu chez le maure de l'ombre et de l'eau – on esquisse une petite sieste mais on ne dort que d'un œil, on n'a pas de temps à perdre. La 2e partie du trajet sera plus longue que la première. Il ne faut pas arriver trop tard. Nous ferons nos adieux au maure, à la petite fille et nous voilà partis.

Nous nous rapprochons de la mer et souvent nous avons à traverser des ruisseaux, des petites rivières que des petits bois de laurier rose nichés dans leur lit, signalent de loin. [**8-b**] Quelques unes paraissent profondes ; comment pourrons nous les traverser. Notre guide Bajonna nous explique que toutes sont ensablées à leur embouchure en ce temps de l'année – ce que nous aurions du deviner à l'absence de courant, et que nous rapprochant de celle nos bêtes en auront à peine jusqu'au ventre. Ainsi se passent les choses en effet et nous passons les « fleuves à pied sec » – deux heures se passent. De la tête de la caravane on entend l'exclamation aqua ! aqua ! C'est un puits. On [va descendre (mots rayés)] faire halte et boire un peu ; il est 3 heures peut-être. Il fait chaud, on a soif. Le puits est profond, l'eau basse. Un maure y descend en s'accrochant aux pierres ; il reparaît, la [**8-c**] cruche pleine et l'on boit une eau fraîche mais un peu trouble. Cependant je m'étais abrité sous un buisson élevé où déjà sans doute on s'était maintes fois assis à en juger par les débris de toute sorte qui jonchaient le sol. J'étais à rêver....nous voilà loin d'Europe, de France, de Paris,...ici rien de banal...lieux presqu'inexplorés et je jouissais de la sensation que donne l'idée « d'une source inconnue où l'on puise le premier » comme dit Lucrèce. Hélas un fragment de journal jauni git à terre. Il semble avoir servi à contenir quelque provision de bouche, à moins qu'il n'ait servi à quelque autre usage... J'y lis en gros caractère, Le Figaro!!! 23 juillet, supplément littéraire ; ce supplément ne doit pas être vendu à part. Du 23 juillet, et [**8-d**] nous sommes le 10 août. Il n'y a que 17 jours que cela a paru.... Le Figaro. C'est bien lui ; hélas ! Quelle chute...et comme cela nous ramène à la modestie. Oui soyons modeste et n'oublions pas que c'est le Figaro, le Figaro hélas ! Qui nous représente surtout à l'étranger...dans la gare de Charring Cross, comme dans tous les patios de Séville, à Peterbourg, comme dans les déserts du Tetuan !... J'emporterai le fragment sali, je lui donnerai une place dans mon album et je le regarderai quelquefois... avec mélancolie.

Je me lève et je me rapproche du groupe des buveurs d'eau, qui se partagent un melon d'eau. Sur le tertre où ils sont [pris place (mots rayés)] assis toutes les places sont occupées. Un des maures du roi, s'en aperçoit ; il s'approche de mon [**9-a**] fils et lui frappant doucement sur l'épaule, il lui dit « le père n'est pas assis » en espagnol. Mon fils se lève et je m'assieds à sa place. Scène de mœurs arabes, fort édifiante en somme et qui montre bien que même si nous sommes chez les Barbaresques nous ne sommes pas chez les Barbares.

Nous voilà de nouveau en route et le chemin nous écarte peu à peu de la mer que bientôt nous perdons de vue ; à droite un petit lac où il y a une foule d'oiseaux sauvages. B. prend le fusil d'un des maures de l'empereur qui nous accompagne. Le coup part, l'oiseau fuit...et n'est pas blessé. Tant mieux, me dis-je *in petto*. En voilà un qui pourra jouir encore longtemps de sa vie d'oiseau à laquelle [**9-b**] sans doute il tient beaucoup. Bon voyage.

Il est six heures, [cinq et demi (mots rayés)] on commence à songer sérieusement à Tetuan. Où est-il ? On ne peut le voir, il

est caché derrière une montagne allongée, dominée par une sorte
de Cap que surmonte une tour – Tetuan nous restera caché pendant longtemps encore, mais sur la gauche nous apercevons une
plaine qui s'étend jusqu'à la mer. Non loin de celle-ci on aperçoit
2 constructions carrées blanches, l'une plus grande que l'autre. La
2e plus près de nous est la douane. L'autre qui paraît toucher à la
mer est la Tour Martin. C'est là que nous nous embarquerons pour
retourner à Ceuta, si le vent est favorable. Nous arrivons à [9-c]
une sorte de ferme juchée sur une colline que nous contournons.
Nos maures du roi y ont des connaissances. Ils sont montés là, nous
les y avons entendu causer....Ils redescendent en courant et nous
ont bientôt rattrapés.

Nous avançons, nous avançons toujours...quand arriverons
nous ?

Dans une heure...environ – enfin voilà des jardins enclos
dans des murailles de bambou. Une porte ouverte laisse voir
quelquefois une maison de campagne ; on entend des voix dans le
jardin. On commence à rencontrer sur la route des gens qui vont
et qui viennent....La plupart saluent et disent quelques mots à nos
maures....Nous approchons sans doute...heureusement ! Car le jour
baisse et nous ne savons par expérience que par ici la nuit vient
vite. Il ne faut pas [9-d] arriver après la fermeture des portes. Par
précaution l'on envoie en ville un de nos maures. Il part en courant
et disparaît bientôt derrière un de ces murs de bambou qui servent
de clôture aux maisons de campagne. Le pas de nos mulets retentit
en frappant le sol, nous voilà sur une chaussée forte mal pavée,
sans doute et toute défoncée....Mais ce doit être une grande route.
Nous approchons sans aucun doute ; il fait presque nuit. À droite
sur une colline se voient des constructions bizarres, imposantes.
C'est nous dit-on le vieux cimetière maure ; à gauche un mur d'environ 2 mètres de haut laisse passer la tête de petites constructions
isolées, à l'air plutôt sinistre, dont en raison de l'obscurité on ne
distingue pas bien la forme ; c'est le nouveau cimetière maure.

[**10-a**] Enfin nous apercevons un grand mur blanc crénelé, percé d'une porte à plein – surmontée d'une fenêtre carrée. La porte est-elle ouverte ou fermée ; placé à la queue de la caravane je me le demande ! Tout à coup l'on s'arrête ; donc la porte est fermée. Allons-nous coucher dehors – on frappe et l'on parle, au dedans comme au dehors...Il paraît y avoir des difficultés : Tout à coup le volet de la petite fenêtre carrée qui surmonte la porte s'ouvre avec fracas, une lumière paraît, puis la silhouette d'un homme, une voix aigrelette articule quelque chose qui ne me paraît guère favorable à notre cause « chiens de chrétiens, il est trop tard...allez vous coucher... en plein [**10-b**] air, ou quelque chose de semblable sans doute...décidément cela va mal. Un bon lit cependant ferait bien mon affaire après cette rude journée – ...un moment de silence. Tout à coup la porte s'ouvre et nous voilà entrés...nous avions des intelligences dans la place....Le maure était arrivé à temps et quelques *taffetas* avaient leur bouclés les difficultés.

Nous voilà dans une rue pavée, étroite, où l'on ne voit goutte – cependant au bout de quelques pas, sur la droite, une grande porte ouverte, nous laisse voir une vaste pièce éclairée par de nombreuses lampes. C'est une mosquée. Nous avançons toujours dans l'obscurité presque complète dans les petites rues sonores et où l'on rencontre à peine de temps en temps un passant.

[**10-c**] Nous débouchons sur une grande place vide en ce moment... encore une mosquée, ouverte et vivement éclairée, nous rentrons dans l'ombre des petites rues étroites – nous voilà dans une ruelle. Tout à coup la tête de colonne s'arrête. Un petit maure bossu, avec lequel nous ferons plus tard ample connaissance sous le nom de Tach Tach, nous éclaire de sa lanterne. Nous [descendons (mot raye)] quittons nos montures et pénétrant par une petite porte à un seul battant, et plus tôt passé, nous pénétrons dans le patio d'une maison maure....c'est la fonda espagnole.

Oui, nous le reconnaîtrons mieux demain, c'est bien là la maison d'un maure de moyenne aisance. Rien n'a été modifié dans la construction : autour du patio, 4 ou 5 cuartos sans fenêtres. L'un d'eux nous sert de salle à manger.

[**10-d**] Les grandes portes en ont été enlevées au premier étage 4 cuartos, également sans fenêtres ; le seul jour qui y pénètre vient de petites meurtrières pratiquées au dessus de la grande porte verte, à deux battants avec gonds cubiques, comme on les voit partout ici. En dedans ces portes se ferment à l'aide d'un verrou énorme, très primitif. Sur l'un des volets de la grande porte est pratiqué une porte plus petite qui peut s'ouvrir seule à la nuit ; on se demande d'où le jour pourra venir demain matin ; mais en élevant les yeux, j'aperçois le ciel noir constellé d'étoiles brillantes. Le plafond est percé dans l'azotia : c'est par là que vient le jour et aussi la pluie, et cela explique qu'une sorte d'impluvium a été pratique sur le sol du patio. Oui tout est maure ici...jusqu'aux [**11-a**] découpures des portes qui du patio conduisent au 1er étage, et de celle qui du 1e étage conduit à l'azotia. La porte qui du patio conduit sur le corridor qui donne dans la rue possède les mêmes découpures. Seuls les meubles arabes ont disparu, remplacés par de bons gros meubles d'Espagne : ainsi nous aurons des lits, des commodes, des bureaux. Etc., etc., des chaises, des fauteuils et nous ne serons pas obligés pour manger ou pour recevoir notre monde de nous accroupir à l'orientale....Ce qui me gênerait diablement vu la rigidité de mes membres inférieurs.

Le dîner est prêt – nous ferons connaissance avec Madm. Juanna un beau type d'Espagnol brune et plantureuse ; très aimable du reste, [**11-b**] avec Jean, l'hôtelier, son mari, homme excellent ; avec les servantes juives qui se mettent en quatre pour nous être agréables. Enfin avec le petit maure Tach Tach, qui désormais, clopin clopant, nous précédera dans nos pérégrinations à travers la ville, muni d'un grand bâton et fusil, dans la nuit, d'une lanterne...Personnage mixte, un peu mystérieux, ménageant la chèvre et le choux et servant de lien entre Israël, Mahomet et le pape.....un grand diplomate au fond à ce que j'ai pu croire.

Nous étonnons et nous étonnerons toujours, dorénavant les gens d'ici par notre inépuisable appétit... on n'aura jamais vu faire tant de repas et de repas si [**11-c**] copieux! Décidément cette cure à [grand (mot raye)] exercice corporel au grand air, par une température moyenne de 35, à l'ombre est chose à conseiller.....J'y réfléchirai. Un bon petit voyage à Tetuan dans la saison chaude... pourquoi pas?

Nous sommes fatigués et nous allons dormir. À demain les affaires sérieuses.

[**Ms A**] [**3-a**] Il fait très chaud. On s'éponge la figure Mais le sommeil nous prend et l'on dort lourdement – le lendemain matin de bonne heure 7 heures on vient nous dire qu'il y a voir une *noce* dans le quartier juif. Quoique un peu fatigué je me lève et m'habille rapidement espérant voir quelque chose comme ce qu'a peint Delacroix. Je ne devais pas être trompé :

11 août 4ᵉ journée. La noce Juive – le quartier juif – le marche – la ville – maisons des maures.

Naturellement il fait beau, c'est la règle et déjà fort chaud bien qu'il ne soit que 7 heures. Pour se rendre au quartier juif qu'une porte à double battant sépare du reste de la ville. (4000 Juifs), il faut traverser la grande place qui déjà est encombrée de monde et d'animaux, car c'est jour de marché. Il y a un grand mouvement. Partout le costume oriental. Rien ne dépare le tableau si ce n'est nous et nous ne nous regardons pas – on reviendra sur le marché tout à l'heure; actuellement c'est le quartier juif qu'il faut voir. Les Juifs se reconnaissent du premier coup [**3-b**] à leur lévite, et à leur coiffure qui consiste en une petite calotte qu'ils placent sur le derrière de la tête, laissant le front couvert seulement par les cheveux. Ils portent en bandoulière une espèce de Besace de cuir rouge le plus souvent, une sorte de portefeuille. Beaucoup portent un anneau d'argent à l'oreille droite – Mais je crois que quelques Maures le portent aussi. Nous voilà arrivés au quartier des Juifs.

Notre passage n'a produit aucune émotion, nulle part. Les rues étroites, recouvertes d'arcades ça et là, les fenêtres grillées partout – des boutiques petites qui ne diffèrent en rien de celles des arabes. Nous arrivons à la maison où a lieu la fête. Ce sont des gens de moyenne aisance. Nous entrons dans une petite cour pleine de monde. Quelques Européens de l'ambassade espagnole sont là, curieux comme nous. On est les uns sur les autres. L'attention se fixe surtout sur 5 ou 6 femmes juives en costume de gala, qui tiennent une grande place – [3-c] sur la tête une calotte de velours, avec franges dorées, brodées – boucles d'oreille énormes – les cheveux remplacés par une perruque noire uniforme – Les yeux sont beaux en général, la face souvent bouffie et strumeuse – une veste rappelant un peu celle des Toréadors. En velours vert foncé ou bleu foncé, avec Broderies. Une grande jupe en velours même couleur, épaisse, pesante, avec d'énormes Broderies sur un coin de la jupe qui est ouverte au milieu. Au cou un collier de riche apparence portant l'aigle a deux têtes de la maison d'Autriche – un vieux rabbin qui se trouve là et passe peut-être à juste titre pour un savant [?] que le costume est celui que portaient les Juifs quand il y a 3 cent [ans] ils habitaient la Castille. Les Juifs de Tetuan étaient en effet des Juifs venant de Castille d'où ils ont été chassés. Ils parlent tous l'espagnol assez purement dit-on – Ils n'auraient donc pas gardé rancune a leurs persécuteurs puisqu'ils ont gardé le costume (?) la langue, et jusqu'a l'aigle!!! Mais de la cour il faut entrer [3-d] dans la maison ou se passent les choses intéressantes. Nous pénétrons dans une petite pièce également bondée de monde; mais on offre aux Européens la 1e place. On s'écarte pour les laisser passer. Il fait une chaleur étouffante et je ne comprends pas, comment ces malheureux en habit de gala lourd et épais, peuvent supporter cette chaleur là – vraiment elles ont l'air de ne pas s'en douter et restent plutôt *pâles*. La chambre où nous entrons est fort petite. Là encore une 10e de femmes en grand costume assises, d'âges divers, plutôt jeunes qui tiennent une place énorme. Mais l'attention se concentre sur la mariée qui est assise, immobile dans un coin et entourée de 5 [?]Femmes, dont la mère – celle-ci et une autre procède à la coiffure – on applique une sorte de diadème : Mais déjà les autres parties du costume ont été appliquées. Une à une, avec un cérémonial analogue sans doute à celui qu'on a observé pour le placement de la coiffure. Celle-ci consiste en une sorte de diadème enroulé autour de la tête et qui doit tenir bien chaud. Déjà la perruque noire a remplacé les cheveux naturels.

[4-a] L'application, la mise des épingles se fait lentement, pendant le temps qu'on y met un chant monotone, rythmé par un tambour de basque ne cesse de se produire, interrompu seulement de temps en temps par une sorte de gémissement de plainte modulée, que pousse une autre femme (celle ci m'a fait l'effet d'une servante) et qui est d'un grand effet. Tout cela est pénétrant, on se sent transporter plusieurs siècles en arrière – ça fait l'effet d'un rêve.

Mais revenons à la mariée. Pendant ce long supplice elle garde une immobilité systématique – on dirait une figure de cire. Les yeux sont fermés. Aucune expression sans doute ne doit se peindre sur la figure légèrement fardée et sur laquelle on a placé ça et là des mouches. La malheureuse ou bienheureuse fait peine à voir. Doit elle avoir chaud et si une démangeaison lui venait au nez...que faire ? Souffrir. serait-elle répudiée pour avoir gratté [4-b] son nez ? Enfin la cérémonie de l'habillage est finie. Elle se dresse debout et fait quelques pas dans la pièce où on l'a habillée et ou se trouve le lit nuptial. Je remarque qu'elle est petite et qu'elle porte des talons. Arrive le promis qui a l'air d'un grand benêt et qui commet l'incongruité à mes yeux de se présenter là en costume Européen. Redingote de drap, melon sur la tête, le voile blanc sur les épaules, gilet de piqué blanc. Il a les mains enveloppées de je ne sais quelles bandelettes, il passe l'anneau au doigt de la mariée et pendant ce temps un homme âgé, barbu, vêtu lui à l'orientale, prononce je ne sais quelles paroles bizarres, ou je remarque pas mal d'Elouim !! La mariée cependant est toujours à l'état de poupée de cire impassible, immobile, aux yeux clos. Vient ensuite si je ne me trompe la cérémonie du verre plein jusqu'aux bords – le rabbin [**4-c**] y trempe ses lèvres et chante encore quelque chose ; un individu qui l'assiste et a l'air d'un sacristain de synagogue avale la bonne moitié du verre – on dit que c'est contraire au rite, mais il fait si chaud – vient le moment où le verre doit être cassé – mais celui où on a bu est un beau verre tout neuf ; le dit sacristain y substitue plus ou moins habilement un verre ébréché, qu'il projette à terre où il se brise avec fracas. C'est le moment si je ne me trompe de la lecture ou plutôt du *chant*, (car tout se chante) du contrat. Celui-ci est un grand parchemin enluminé, où tout est écrit en hébreu. Sur chaque coin de ce parchemin se voit une main se présentant par la paume et où les 2 derniers doigts accolés l'un à l'autre sont séparés des 2 premiers également accolés, par un écartement de 2 ou 3 centimètres – qu'est ce que cela signifie. J'ai vu de pareilles mains en métal suspendues dans les synagogues de quartier. Mais les doigts n'étaient pas écartés ainsi.

[**4-d**] Pendant tout le temps que cela dure on entend retentir par moments ce gémissement modulé qui fait tant d'effet depuis le commencement de la cérémonie – La mariée disparait, toujours poupée de cire – on l'amène je crois se déshabiller dans la pièce où a lieu l'habillement et où se trouve le lit nuptial dont les rideaux de gaze épaisse sont tirés, on dresse une table où l'on sert des mets bizarres que nous aurons à goûter tout à l'heure, car nous sommes bien et dûment des invités et quand les gens de la famille auront fini, ce qui ne sera pas long, ce sera notre tour, il faudra nous exécuter. Notre tour est venu. Nous prenons place à la table. On nous verse une sorte d'aquardiente, que nous goûtons des lèvres – des œufs durs, des gâteaux – des morceaux de courge confite, et quelques autres singularités de confiserie que nous apprécions diversement. La plus grand partie reste sur l'assiette. Mais nous avons fait notre devoir. Oui notre devoir d'invités et de curieux par une température de 38 à 40.

[5-a] Pendant ce temps la mariée a pris place sur le lit. Son costume est changé – elle occupe le milieu du lit le dos au mur, accroupie à l'orientale. Maintenant elle a les yeux ouverts. Ils sont beaux sans doute – mais tout est obscur sous les rideaux. À sa droite et à sa gauche sont accroupies, comme elle, d'autres femmes, dont la mère à gauche. Chacun de nous passe devant le lit et tend la main à la mère d'abord, puis à la fille en saluant – où est passe le marié – on ne le voit plus ; il semble qu'il n'en soit plus question pour le moment – La cérémonie n'est point terminée ; il y aura bien d'autres réjouissances ; Mais le temps passe et nous avons bien d'autres choses à voir – Il est temps d'aller déjeuner plus sérieusement et d'ailleurs il faut à tout prix sortir de cette chaudière.

[5-b] Nous voilà partis. Nous traversons de nouveau la place. Nous sommes bientôt à l'hôtel ; nous déjeunons rapidement et nous voilà repartis.

Buisson, Jean et Jeanne s'en vont aux emplettes : moi je prends le parti de m'installer devant la pharmacie espagnole ; assis, aussi confortablement que possible, sous une véranda, où se fait habituellement la consultation gratuite : je suis là assis entre le pharmacien, M. X, et le médecin M. X Barada, tous les deux sont au service de l'ambassade espagnole. Ce sont des espagnols issus de Maures : le père et le grand-père portent encore le costume des maures aisés et sont fort aimables, en espagnol. Les 2 enfants ont étudié à Madrid – sont-ils ou non catholiques ?

De mon poste on peut sans avoir par trop chaud, embrasser toute la place qui est enflammée par un soleil brûlant (ça a été dit on, un des plus chauds jours du mois)

[5-c] Comme c'est jour de marché, la distribution des médicaments se fait sur une assez grande échelle – Les juifs seuls viennent prendre les médicaments ou les consultations. Il paraît que les Arabes ne consultent pas ! (Je n'ai rien su ou pu savoir de leurs Talebs – Je regarde surtout ce qui se passe sur la place – d'abord le lieu, puis le contenu – En face la porte ouverte d'une mosquée – en

face toujours mais vers la droite le palais, surmonté d'une sorte de tour carrée, recouvert d'un toit à tuiles vertes, rappelant ce qu'on voit à Grenade. Dans le lointain la ville qui s'étend vers la Kasbah, les murs qui rattachent celle-ci à l'enceinte – enfin les montagnes qui forment le fond du tableau – à droite la porte du consulat qui ne se distingue des autres que par l'inscription. Dépassant la crête du mûr, un dôme surmonté d'une croix. On a fait monter ce dôme assez haut afin qu'on le voie bien. C'est l'église du couvent de je ne sais quels *pères* espagnols que nous allons visiter demain et qui vivent là, depuis la guerre, sous la [5-d] protection du consul. La porte du quartier des juifs est dans l'angle qui suit, dans le carré que forme la place, le côté où s'ouvre le consulat avec le côté où se trouve la pharmacie. Sur le côté du carré situé à ma gauche, s'ouvrent 3 où 4 rues parmi lesquelles une où j'irai plus tard et vous conduit immédiatement dans un des caravansérails de la ville, le plus grand je pense. Un côté de ce caravansérail qui forme un grand carré, constitue un des côtés de la grande place – à côté de la pharmacie coule une fontaine ou viennent puiser et s'abreuver un tas de gens, Juifs et Maures et aussi nombre de Kabyles venus de la campagne à l'occasion du marché et qui disparaîtront demain.

Ce qu'on voit sur la place : Cela m'intéresse plus : L'orient n'est pas dépassé par l'Europe. Tous juifs d'Afrique ou musulmans vendant des poules, des ânes parmi lesquels des microscopiques qu'on pourrait peut-être emporter dans les bras. Il y a des gens de la ville, il y a des gens des environs. Quelques uns sont venus.

[6-a] sur des chameaux que l'on voit au nombre de 8 ou 10 – ça tient de la place un chameau – dans le caravansérail d'à côté. Les jeunes maures avec le fez, les maures avec le turban ; les arabes nomades ou campagnards qui ont plutôt l'air de bandits avec le burnous. Les femmes couvertes d'un grand chapeau de paille, et le burnous avec la fente traditionnelle qui laisse voir les yeux – quelques unes laissent tout voir ce sont les Laides – elles ont une sorte de bosse dans le dos : c'est sans doute un paquet caché par le

burnous : La preuve c'est que le paquet est quelquefois un enfant. Dans ce cas une fente est pratiquée au dos du burnous, laquelle laisse passer le tronc et la tête du bébé. Toute sont femmes du peuple je pense. Je n'ai pas vu une seule « dame » se promener là. Mais on m'a dit que dans les rues marchandes on avait pu en voir – tout cela s'agite froidement [6-b] sans grand bruit et partout résonne la langue gutturale – un cercle s'est formé sur un coin de la place ; au milieu un homme s'agite et parle. Je m'approche malgré qu'il faille traverser la place en plein soleil pensant qu'il s'agit de quelque mangeur de serpents ; c'est peut être de quelque chose comme cela qu'il s'agit : mais je n'ai pas le courage d'attendre jusqu'à la fin du boniment. Il fait trop chaud. Il m'avait été facile de comprendre d'ailleurs que notre homme ne ferait autre chose que ce que nous voyons souvent sur nos places de Paris : « allons MM du courage à la poche, faites la somme ! Croyez vous que je vais vous montrer ceci et cela pour 5 sous, pour 10 sous – fi donc – etc etc – et les acolytes assis a l'orientale dans le cercle, autour du charlatan font force musique avec leurs guitares et les tambourines pour suggérer au public la générosité et la curiosité : ce sera peut être [6-c] encore long : j'aime mieux battre en retraite vers mon observatoire ou je trouverai de l'ombre et un verre d'eau fraiche. Jean, Jeanne, Buisson et Bayonna arrivent des rues commerçantes de la ville où ils ont vu des merveilles ; ils sont cuites : il est temps d'aller redéjeuner – partons. Au revoir MM. les médecins et pharmaciens. Ce dernier nous montre quelques bonnes photographies que nous achetons.

Le déjeuner ne présente rien de spécial. On est fort gai et fort content de tout ce que l'on voit. Il n'y a qu'un petit point noir qu'on n'ose s'avouer. Pas de nouvelles, impossibilité d'en avoir et d'en faire parvenir. J'ai prévenu Augustine que cet état durerait 4 jours. Ce sera certainement plus, même en allant vite – nous devions le soir même avoir une bien agréable surprise. Le gouverneur nous ferait savoir que d'Algesiras à l'aide du télégraphe militaire, on avait

transmis 2 dépêches de Madame Charcot – bonnes nouvelles :
Le ciel de Tetuan [6-d] nous en paraît plus beau, l'air plus léger,
la chaleur moindre, et tout ce que l'on voit plus intéressant ; Ce
que c'est que de nous et comme ils ont raison ceux qui disent que
tout est en nous...à la condition toutefois qu'il vienne qq chose du
dehors, bien entendu !!

On prolonge le repas, on cause, on reçoit des marchands qui
apportent les achats ou en proposent. Pendant ce temps le temps
de la grande chaleur passe. Alors arrive le consul d'Espagne qui
aura la complaisance de nous mener à travers les rues de la ville
visiter la maison de 2 maures riches, comme on dit et qui nous
attendent chez eux. Ses 2 demoiselles l'accompagnent, on a bientôt
fait connaissance avec Jeanne. Il est convenu que ces demoiselles
rendront visite aux dames ; tandis que nous, bien entendu nous ne
pénétrerons pas dans les appartements intimes, c'est bien clair.
Nous pénétrons dans le dédale ; l'avantage des rues étroites est
palpable, dans [7-a] ce climat, dans cette saison. On a de l'ombre ;
il fait presque frais. Souvent la rue est couverte par une arcade,
d'autrefois par une treille ; dans les éclaircies on voit le ciel ; il
fait très clair partout et l'on ne se plaint pas de l'ombre grand
Dieu. Quelquefois au bout d'une rue l'apparition d'un minaret,
cela de la Kasbah surmontant son rocher fait le meilleur effet :
à droite et à gauche [on ne peut arrêter ?] les yeux. Partout les
marchands à l'air grave et le plus souvent distingué, même quand
il s'agit de cordonniers, de forgerons, d'épiciers, d'armuriers, etc.
accroupis dans leurs petites boutiques où fourmillent les objets
de vente : ils nous regardent d'un air distrait et se moquent de
nous probablement. Un vieux bouquiniste est en train de lire un
grand livre qui est peut-être le Coran. On fait [7-b] mine de lui
vouloir acheter quelque chose ; il ne détourne même pas la tête et
continuant à lire il fait comprendre par geste que nous l'impor-
tunons et qu'il ne vendra rien. Ça et là une porte de mosquée
ouverte. Une planche en travers sur laquelle s'accoude un tas de

gamins, enferme l'entrée, mais le regard plonge aisément dans le péristyle où siège le bassin des ablutions, puis dans le sanctuaire toujours construit sur le modèle, en raccourci bien entendu, de la cathédrale de Cordoue. J'ai même plusieurs fois aperçu dans le fin fond le Mihrab ! Des lampes sont pendues a la vue (nous les avons vues allumées plusieurs fois, dans la nuit, en particulier le jour de notre arrivée) et hélas aussi, quelquefois quelques unes de ces grosses boules brillantes argentées dont les bourgeois sans goût de notre pays ornent [7-c] nos jardins — nous nous arrêtons quelquefois regardant tout cela curieusement. Personne ne proteste. Cependant quelquefois un vieux cagot accroupi dans un coin, nous regarde avec un certain air menaçant qui montre bien que si l'on bravait la consigne on le ferait une affaire. Non loin des mosquées quelquefois une porte toujours ouverte donne accès dans un lieu où se trouve un certain nombre de cabinets d'aisance, avec porte, et trou à fleur de tinette — une place est réservée à une piscine dans laquelle l'arabe monte pour se laver à grande eau les mollets. L'eau coule partout dans ces lieux-la et cela ne sent pas par trop mauvais.

Mais nous voilà bientôt arrivés chez l'un de nos « Maures riches » — les boutiques cessent d'exister un instant ; nous enfilons un couloir comme nous en avons tant vus ; [7-d] et enfin devant une porte que rien ne distingue des autres ; je remarque même que la rue est en ce lieu, aussi mal pavée — des espèces de gros cailloux, avec une sorte de rigole au milieu comme à Algesiras et à Ceuta — cela vous coupe les pieds — et aussi peu entretenue que partout ailleurs. Des eternes d'ânes et de mulet et des toiles d'araignées sur la façade partout il peut s'en [?] — Cela me parait être la règle ; rien ne distingue la porte du riche (c'est prudence sans doute) et en parcourant les rues les seules choses qui attirent l'attention par leur ornementation, en dehors des boutiques, ce sont les portes des mosquées et de temps en temps de charmantes fontaines polychromes qui font le meilleur effet dans les carréfours.

Mais j'en reviens à notre visite. On frappe, la porte s'ouvre et nous voilà dans une antichambre [8-a] qui respire déjà l'aisance. Le parquet comme les parois à hauteur de main sont fait de ces mosaïques de faïence qui rappellent ce qu'on voit à Grenade. Il y a des bancs également en mosaïque à droite et à gauche – s'ouvre une 2e porte et nous voilà dans le patio, richement décoré de la même façon. C'est frais c'est charmant, c'est d'une propreté irréprochable : l'eau coule sans cesse dans une petite vasque située au centre où s'agite une eau limpide. Le sol est comme les murs jusqu'à hauteur de main (les colonnes plus haut) pavé de ces mosaïques charmantes : on n'ose pas marcher là dessus avec des bottes : nos hôtes ont des babouches – un trou aux 4 coins du patio laisse passer le tronc d'un bel oranger qui s'élance vers l'azotia pour y trouver le jour qui cependant ne fait pas défaut – Les chambres sont fermées par ces grandes portes [8-b] à deux battants avec lesquelles nous avons fait connaissance déjà à la fonda espagnole – quelques unes sont ouvertes on n'y voit aucun ornement – çà et là seulement des glaces de tout style, véritable collection. Ou encore des pendules de tous les genres : il y a des *cathédrales* ; beaucoup viennent sans doute du Boulevard St Denis. Cela tranche remarquablement avec l'ornementation locale qui est très fine, très délicate et dont on peut admirer la variété sur les portes grandes ou petites, où les fleurs et les ornements de tout genre sont peints du meilleur goût – Les murs au dessus de la fayence sont blancs : mais on nous montre que dans la saison d'hiver on les recouvre en partie d'étoffes aux couleurs voyantes, dont la disposition rappelle ces étoffes [8-c] drapées qu'on peint sur les murs de nos cathédrales restaures suivant le style d'époque, et qui peut-être dans le temps existaient en réalité et non pas seulement en peinture.

Les demoiselles pénètrent chez les dames. Nous nous fouillons partout où nous avons accès d'un œil scrutateur. Je crois que l'on nous attendait et très certainement on nous attendait – Cependant un émoi feint sans doute, une surprise simulée a eu lieu à notre entrée. Une dame d'un certain âge et qui m'a paru belle s'est enfuie rapidement mais non sans nous montrer sa face ; seules sont restées sans vergogne 4 ou 5 négresses fort belles du reste, au bras et jambes nues, le corps vêtu **[8-d]** légèrement d'une étoffe claire : elles n'appartiennent pas sans doute à la religion où l'on se cache. Il y a comme toujours un premier étage avec balcon qui reproduit à peu prés là disposition du bas : là on n'a pas accès paraît il ; ce sont les appartements intimes : partout je cherche un certain lieu qui m'intéresse comme hygiéniste : L'instinct me conduit – Là l'eau coule à terre, on n'y peut entrer sans doute sans des socques – le sol est en mosaïque de fayence ainsi que les parois – pas de siège – à terre seulement un trou qui m'a paru étroit. Il faut être habile – mais les arabes le sont sans doute de ce côté : ils font tout accroupis. C'est une perfection, un paradis au point de la vision et de l'odorat.

Notre hôte qui nous a admirablement reçu parle espagnol ; il est temps de se retirer – ces dames reviennent et ont beau jeu à constater des merveilles : on se serre la main et l'on se dirige chez le 2e maure riche.

[9-a] On rentre dans le labyrinthe des rues et l'œil ne se rassasie pas de réponses à droite et à gauche – il y a le quartier des cordonniers, celui des armuriers, des marchands d'étoffes, etc. Ou tout au moins cette classification existe en principe – Les peintres sur bois qui font de belles armoires illustrées d'une façon intéressante sont nombreux ; Le travail est quelquefois très fin ; Les tons sont criards – je voudrais bien avoir de ces ouvriers là pour peindre mes portes et mes plafonds à Neuilly.

Nous voilà arrivés chez notre 2e maure. La porte n'en diffère plus que l'autre fois : on entre : même antichambre. La disposition du patio est un peu différente. Toujours le patio à colonnes, la fayence, et la vasque centrale. Mais en haut l'œil est arrêté par une sorte de coupole dont l'ornementation en stalactites rappelle l'Alhambra. On me dit que le propriétaire est un **[9-b]** moderniste et que sa maison est moderne : l'ornementation cependant est [?] emprunts étranges – comme le patio n'est pas à ciel ouvert, par une conséquence logique on n'y a pas mis d'arbres ; mais par contre par une heureuse disposition, de nombreuses fenêtres largement ouvertes, et presque juxtaposées, percent tout un des côtés du patio et laissent voir un jardin d'abord, puis la campagne qui n'en finit plus. La maison est placée près des remparts, du côté par où nous sortirons après demain – on découvre la plaine où coule le rio martin, à distance 2 ou 3 lieues peut-être la douane blanche et carrée, un peu plus loin la tour Martin où nous nous embarquerons si Dieu le veut et enfin la mer qui nous portera à Ceuta.

J'examine avec attention le petit jardin sur lequel s'ouvrent les baies dont je viens de parler. Il est extrêmement soigné. **[9-c]** Les allées surélevées sont pavées de fayences en mosaïque bleu, blanc, mauves et vert, comme partout ailleurs – entre les allées les carrés où l'on voit la terre toujours arrosée contiennent des orangers, des grenadiers. etc. Pas de palmiers – des espèces de constructions de bois en treilles, portant le jasmin qui ne sait pas se tenir seul. C'est un jardin boudoir, très amusant.

Une sorte de pièce, en galerie, sépare les fenêtres du patio. Là je vois 2 beaux lits en cuivre, venant probablement d'Angleterre. On n'a pas l'air d'y coucher. C'est peut-être un objet de curiosité. L'on doit coucher sur les coussins bas en forme de divan que l'on voit dans toutes les autres chambres : ici la collection de glaces et de pendules est des plus riches ; c'est affreux. Mais nous collectionnons les bibelots des autres ; pourquoi ne collectionnerait-t-on pas les nôtres. Je ne désespère pas de voir quelque pot de chambre à fleurs sur une étagère. **[9-d]** même cérémonie pour les dames – mêmes adieux courtois et nous allons rentrer chez nous enchantés de ce que nous avons vu.

Nous voilà de retour à l'hôtel ; nous dinons de bon cœur. – pas de mets arabes. Pas de kouskousou mais une bonne nourriture

espagnole – Il était arrangé que le soir nous irions au café maure
entendre de la musique – Nous voilà partis à travers les rue noires
comme un four. Tach Tach nous précède avec une lanterne. Nous
rencontrons quelques promeneurs çà et là avec une lanterne. Pas
beaucoup. Tout le monde est chez soi – on entend chanter par ici
par là avec accompagnement de guitare et de tambourins. Nous
voilà arrivés en face du café : je ne sais ce qui se passe : il est de
mauvaise humeur. Il n'a personne chez lui, ferme les volets de la
boutique et sa porte à notre nez et barbe – nous voilà assis sur un
banc nous consultant sur ce qu'il y à faire pour employer bien la
soirée. Pendant ce temps passé par là un de *ces fous* errants dont
nous avons rencontrés plusieurs **[10-a]** sur le marché ce matin, qui
vociféraient. Celui-ci est tranquille, il grommelle je ne sais quoi. On
lui donne quelques sous ; il dit merci probablement et disparait dans
l'obscurité d'une voûte. Cependant il a été convenu qu'on enverrait
prendre du thé dans un autre endroit et que nous ferions venir
les musiciens à l'hôtel. Nous retrouvons ce thé aromatisé et dans
lequel nagent cette fois des herbes vertes, que nous avons appris
à connaître sur la frontière marocaine. Nous reprenons le chemin
de l'hôtel. Les musiciens au nombre de 4 nous accompagnent. Ils
s'installent dans le patio. Il y a un violiniste, c'est le chef ; on me
dit que c'est le caporal de Tetuan. Il joue de son instrument comme
on joue de la basse avec une grande habilité. Il y a un guitariste :
une grande mandoline plate qu'il ne fait qu'accorder du matin et
soir, qui a de grosses cordes et qui rend des sons rauques ; Il [y a]
[10-b] un « tambour de basque » ? Enfin une espèce de tambour
en forme de toupie sur lequel on tappe avec la face palmaire des
doigts, des 2 mains et que je crois avoir déjà [vu] entre les mains
des gens de Ceuta – les voilà gravement accroupis. Le chef a un
Burnous et un Turban blanc, ainsi que le joueur de guitare. Les
autres portent le Fez. On s'accorde en prélude ; vient le chant ; ils
ont l'air de s'encourager les uns les autres : enfin les voilà partis.
Ils paraissent bien savoir leur affaire. Voilà un couplet, 2 couplets ;

ça n'en finit plus. Chaque couplet se termine brusquement alors qu'on s'y attend le moins. Je cherche à comprendre – l'harmonie bien entendu – pas les paroles : je ne comprends pas bien. J'aime mieux les Sévillanes – On prend un autre morceau – c'est à peu près la même chose :... je me sens un peu fatigué et sans rien dire à la société ; [10-c] sournoisement, je monte me coucher enchanté de ma journée.

12ᵉ août – 5ᵉ journée

3ᵉ jour à Tetuan. : comme toujours il fait beau quand le matin le jour pénètre à travers la fente de ma porte. Il s'agit ce matin d'aller visiter dans le quartier juif, une maison de riche Juif : l'école et tout ce qu'il peut y avoir de curieux par là.

La maison du Juif – qui entre parenthèse est un vieux filou – ne diffère pas essentiellement de celle du maure. C'est la même construction générale – Patio à colonnes – un étage – mais c'est moins luxueux et c'est plus sale. Pas de faïence sur le sol, ni sur les murs – on nous offre je ne sais quelle boisson alcoolique et je ne sais quelles confiseries – Il cherche à nous endoctriner pour des achats – nous ne nous laissons pas prendre. Une des filles met sur elle, pour le montrer à Jeanne, un costume semblable à celui que nous avons vu hier matin à la noce.

[10-d] On nous chippe quelques consultations – Tous ces gens là sont eczémateux, arthritiques, bouffis, strumeux – 2 enfants de quelques mois. Ils ont dans l'aine des ganglions indurés et enflammés. Cela me parait être des accidents de la circoncision.

Le vieux juif devrait nous offrir la moindre des choses pour ces consultations multiples. Il n'en veut rien faire. Je me venge en écrivant dessus – *gratuit* – Il s'en fiche pas mal.

Nous nous rendons à l'école où l'on enseigne le français et l'espagnol ; c'est une école juive soutenue par une société inter-nationale où les français dominent sans doute : les professeurs ont été élèves en France ; j'essaye de leur faire dire quelque chose qui montre qu'ils se rattachent par un lien sentimental au pays où ils ont vécu et dont ils enseignent la langue : *rien*, ce sont des *heimatlosen* – pas de patrie. La patrie partout – Il y a des garçons et des filles. [11-a] Jamais les maures ne viennent à ces écoles ; bien que la chose soit possible. À ce propos je dirai que j'ai désiré voir une école arabe ; il n'y a pas eu moyen ; l'école ne siégeait pas ; c'était jour de congé – Du quartier juif nous nous rendons au consulat d'Espagne pour y faire nos visites ; et par la même occasion nous nous rendons chez les Turcs qui nous font voir leur église et nous montrent leur bibliothèque Arabe. Après quelques tournées dans les rues, retour à la maison pour déjeuner.

Il est entendu que je donnerai quelques consultations : on m'en à prié. Quelques personnes sont recommandées par le consul, ou par M. Alvans l'envoyé militaire inépuisable dans la complaisance ou par Bajonna.

Voilà les malades qui arrivent. Il en vient 5 ou 6, tous juifs. Ils s'accumulent dans le patio. J'en croque un qui [11-b] offre un bel exemple de Parkinson. Rien de bien intéressant au point de vue de la nosographie ; mais tous sont des nerveux – hier sur la place on m'a montré un juif qui était resté muet dit-on pendant toute son enfance et qui a fini par parler. Était ce un hystérique ?

La consultation est finie ; il faut encore voir la ville afin d'en emporter avec moi une empreinte visuelle difficile à effacer – chemin faisant, engagés dans une des rues les plus habitées, nous entendons à distance une sorte de chant confus à la fois et monotone : ce sont des voix d'hommes. Ils apparaissent ; c'est un cortège ils sont une centaine environ ; ils marchent vite ; on les dirait pressés « les morts vont vite ». De fait c'est un enterrement. Le mort est porté sur une espèce de lit-cage, nu dans un suaire blanc qui le cache en entier la tête y compris. Il me semble que personne autour ne bouge et ne salue ; nous ne saluons [11-c] pas non plus : ce n'est pas la mode ici. Laissons passer le cortège nous le retrouverons dans un instant, au cimetière.

Il était convenu que ce soir vers 4 ou 5 heures nous nous rendrions à l'invitation d'un Maure riche [que nous avions visité déjà hier dans sa maison de ville (mots rayés)] client du D^r X : il nous attendait dans sa maison de campagne située peut-être à un kilomètre de la ville. Il n'était pas sans intérêt de pénétrer dans une de ces enceintes à bambou impénétrable à l'œil, que nous avons remarquées en si grand nombre le soir de notre arrivée à Tetuan, et puis après la vie à la ville il était bon de voir ce que pouvait bien être la vie à la campagne. Nous sortons par la porte [lacune en texte], celle qu'on nous avait autrefois fermée au nez. Ce n'est pas le chemin le plus court pour aller à la maison de campagne, mais nous n'y perdrons rien ; nous aurions à côtoyer les murs bas du cimetière, et nous y verrons de loin, car aux chiens de chrétiens, le lieu saint est fermé, l'enterrement du brave homme que nous venons de voir passer. C'est l'occasion de revoir aussi en plein jour et plus tranquillement le cimetière ancien [11-d] composé de monuments funéraires qui s'étagent en dehors du mur d'enceinte, sur la colline que couronne la Kasbah : Plusieurs de ces tombes sont importantes par la grandeur et par le style ; les plus grandes sont sur le sommet de la colline et se profilent sur le ciel : Il y a ça et là des gens qui semblent y prier – on dit que ces tombeaux sont ceux des premiers maures d'importance qui chassés de Grenade sont venus se réfugier à Tetuan. Le cimetière moderne est de l'autre côté de la route – on y chercherait en vain des monuments rappelant ceux qu'on voit dans les cimetières Turcs, à Constantinople ; Il s'agit simplement ici pour les plus pauvres de pierres juxtaposées formant un ovale et circonscrivant la terre où le mort a été enfoui – d'autrefois c'est un petit mur blanche à la chaux, sorte de clôture qui enceint un petit jardin où une main pieuse cultive qq arbustes ; rien de monumental, tant cela est pauvre : mais l'intention est évidemment excellente. Nous voyons tout cela sans nous déranger. Le mur qui limite le champ où nous ne pouvons pénétrer ayant à peine la hauteur de 2 mètres. Dans le [12-a] lointain, nous voyons enterrer notre homme. Toujours des chants : quelques feuillages. Il me semble que chacun vient à son tour mettre quelque chose, un peu de terre sans doute, sur la tombe – c'est bientôt fait – Ils disparaissent les uns après les autres et bientôt il ne reste plus personne. C'est vite fait. Il y a cependant de la piété pour les morts. Je vois des femmes qui rodent autour des tombes que je décrivais tout à l'heure – Mais il faut nous rendre chez notre maure : c'est à 8 ou 10 minutes plus loin le long des murs de la ville ; nous suivons un chemin bordé à droite et à gauche par des murailles de bambou semblable à celles que nous avons vues maintes fois déjà. Enfin on nous montre une porte que Tach Tach connait et c'est ouvert : c'est une porte en bois encadrée dans un ouvrage de maçonnerie. C'est là. Le jardin est assez peu soigné : ce sont des orangers, des grenadiers, des châssis qui supportent des jasmins. Les arbres sont élevés en manière [12-b] de chaussée au dessus du sol que des conduits d'eau doivent maintenir humides ; Nous arrivons à la maison où on nous attend. Maison carrée peinte à la chaux en blanc cru avec azotea, comme c'est la règle ; un seul étage – en avant une terrasse pavée des mosaïques que vous savez ; autour de la terrasse règne un banc également recouvert de fayence cloisonnée ; cela a du rester très joli, très cossu et bien facile à rendre propre – mais cela est négligé – de cette terrasse qui n'est pas élevée au dessus du sol de plus de 2 mètres on domine cependant toute l'étendue du jardin – auprès de la maison, un puits – Cette maison dans laquelle nous pénétrons plus tard, est fort soignée à l'intérieur ; elle est revêtue de mosaïques comme les maisons des riches visitées hier. Mais ici pas de meubles. Ces Messieurs n'habitent pas là. Ils se contentent sans doute d'y venir prendre l'air de temps en temps dans la saison chaude.

[12-c] Une servante juive parait cependant y vivre – c'est elle qui prépare tout ce qu'il faut faire pour le thé qu'on va nous servir dans un instant. Notre hôte et son ami sont assis près de nous ; le plus vieux prépare lui-même le thé aromatisé que nous connaissons

déjà ; il fourre dans la théière des feuilles d'une plante fraîche qu'on ne lui connait pas. Nous buvons ce thé avec plaisir ; 3 tasses et des gâteaux à l'avenant. Le plus jeune de nos hôtes est un homme de haut taille, mince à figure fort distinguée, à costume très élégant : il parle bien l'espagnol. Il s'éloigne, va cueillir discrètement quelques fleurs dans le jardin et en compose un bouquet qu'il offre à Jeanne très galamment et très discrètement. Il ressemble à mon ami Mohammed Beinam. Je voudrais bien communiquer avec lui ; mais il ne sait pas le Français et moi je ne sais pas l'Espagnol....ni l'arabe – Dans un coin nous voyons le fameux Tac Tac, qui profitant d'un moment propice se passe successivement 3 ou 4 tasses [12-d] de thé qu'on ne l'a pas invité à prendre. Mais je le crois fort bien avec la Juive.

Avant de quitter ce lieu fort agréable nous montons sur l'azotea pour voir le paysage et surtout assister au coucher de soleil derrière la Kasbah. Nous voyons le cimetière vieux, qui je ne sais pourquoi attire toujours le regard, entrer peu à peu dans l'ombre. Je jette un coup d'œil sur le cimetière Juif, qui n'est pas loin et où l'accumulation de tombes blanches fait – au loin l'effet de linge blanches qu'on sèche en plein air.

Nous regagnons la ville à pied avec nos hôtes : nous rentrons par la grande porte, la principale, sur le côté où les fortifications plus modernes, semblent ancienne blanche et préparée – Une chaussée mal pavée et toute bousculée y conduit. Nous suivons une rue tortueuse où il n'y a pas de boutiques – une fontaine ornementale et polychrome se présente en face de la porte – un peu plus loin je remarque une fenêtre ouverte, mais [13-a] fermée d'une grille de bois cloisonné où sont suspendus une foule de petits scapulaires semblables à ceux que portent nos restes chrétiennes – c'est un petit sanctuaire où brûle une lampe à clarté douteuse ; à droite s'ouvre une rue tortueuse également sans boutique – décidément ce n'est pas le quartier commerçant – c'est par cette rue que s'éloignent nos hôtes après nous avoir serré la main – pendant ce temps la nuit s'est faite; elle se fait ici avec rapidité. Nous sommes sur la grande place et nous regagnons l'hôtel où le diner nous attend.

Aujourd'hui encore nous n'avons pas perdu de temps et nous connaissons un peu Tetuan qu'il nous faudra quitter demain.

Après diner nombreuses visites d'adieu – l'une d'elles a un caractère important. Nous voyons apparaître tout à coup la plus belle lanterne à verres de couleur que nous ayons vu encore; elle est suivie par le maure du consulat, qui s'avance lentement d'un air imposant, une [13-b] canne dans celle de ses mains qui ne porte pas la majestueuse lanterne. Il annonce pompeusement le consul d'Espagne qui apparaît bientôt demeurant suivi de ses deux filles. Je ne sais pas pourquoi cette promenade aux lanternes me rappelle le 2e acte d'obéron et la charmante musique de marche, chants et accompagnements, qui marquent le pas de la patrouille.

Les adieux se préparent on se fait quelques un différent à demain matin!

Cependant quelques gouttes de pluie tombent dans le patio – Le temps change; le vent nous sera-t-il favorable pourrons nous partir par mer ou faudra-t-il refaire à mulet les 12 ou 14 heures de marche!! Bajonna prétend que les pronostics sont favorables – La barque est arrivée de Ceuta. Elle nous attend là bas, près du fort Martin – est ce par là que nous irons – Nous verrons bien cela demain; qu'y faire d'ailleurs. [13-c] Allons nous coucher et dormons ferme.

13 août Le lendemain matin vers 6h1/2 j'ouvre les yeux et je vois le soleil. Je me lève et suis bientôt prêt. Je monte sur l'azotea d'où l'on a une vue magnifique. Il fait du vent – est-ce du bon vent?

Je prends un dessin de ce qu'on voit de la ville du côté de la Kasbah – le château, la grande mosquée et son minaret, puis une foule de petites mosquées : toutes portent ce matin un drapeau rouge qui flotte au vent. C'est fête aujourd'hui; c'est vendredi – on a orné toute la nuit, et de très bonne heure j'ai entendu un coup de canon. On entend aussi les petits concerts qui se font à la porte des mosquées – nous verrons cela tout à l'heure.

La tour carrée du château, couverte de ses briques vertes, fait d'ici un bon effet. Hier nous avons visité l'intérieur qui est à moitié ruiné, mais ou il y a de bien beaux restes. Des [? moustiques] partout; des capillaires et des scolopendres plein les fontaines. **[13-d]** Le patio est occupé par je ne sais quel fabricant. Hier quand nous sommes entrés, sous la porte était accroupi le gouverneur entouré d'un certain nombre de ses agents. Ils paraissaient compter de l'argent en plein air ou peu s'en faut. En même temps dans le fond d'une cour j'aperçois un fidèle, qui à genoux fait des gesticulations étranges; il fait une prière mouvementée.

Tout cela me revient à l'esprit en faisant mon croquis; je me retourne de l'autre côté – on voit la place et le quartier juif. Je prendrais bien encore un croquis car je suis en verve. Mais le temps presse il faut aller déjeuner.

Cependant les mules sont préparées sur la grande place – Les unes portent des provisions, les autres nous porteront. Nos amis de Tetuan nous attendent là – quelques uns nous accompagneront jusqu'à la barque – adieu, au revoir – la cavalcade s'ébranle – nous sortons de la ville par le côté que le bombardement a ruiné et que nous avons visité déjà. **[14-a]** Partout des masures qui tombent en ruines. C'est morne et triste; cela a été ruiné il y a près de 20 ans. On n'a rien réparé depuis. Une porte se présente : nous la franchissons et à partir de là nous suivons une vieille muraille d'aspect très pittoresque. Nous voilà dans la plaine qui conduit à la mer. Tetuan se présente à nous d'une façon pittoresque. À chaque instant je me retourne pour la voir encore; elle s'éloigne, s'éloigne et on l'embrasse de mieux en mieux; nous voilà près de la maison de campagne où nous étions hier. Au détour d'un chemin Tach Tach apparait; il vient nous faire ses adieux – La campagne à mesure que nous avançons devient de plus en plus aride – c'est à un moment un désert de sable – Cependant le Rio Martin est une assez grande rivière – nous voilà arrivés à la douane – nous sommes partis à 10 h il est près de 1 heure nous avons encore 1/2 heure de chemin pour arriver [**14-b**] à la tour Martin où nous attend la barque de Bajonna. On embarque quatre hommes d'équipage : Le vent est bon – nos 2 maures du roi reviennent à Ceuta avec nous. Le vent est favorable. Il enfle bientôt la voile – nous voilà partis. Il est temps de déjeuner.

Mais on jette encore un regard sur Tetuan qui nous a été si hospitalière – on la voit encore se profiler en blanc sur le fond noir des montagnes ; là est le grand minaret, ici la grotte de [lacune en texte], la Kasbah juchée sur sa colline et à côté le vieux cimetière ; adieu fille de Grenade, nous allons bientôt rendre à ta mère une pieuse visite.

Revenons aux choses pratiques. Donc le vent est bon ; Si cela continue nous pourrons attendre Ceuta dans 3 ou 4 heures. Mais cela continuera-t-il ? Qui le sait ! Il faut toujours compter avec l'élément perfide…false lethe water – Mais on a faim et pendant que le bateau file gentiment on éventre les sacs à provisions : il y a des assiettes des plats, des serviettes des fourchettes, rien n'y manque : [**14-c**] Mme Juanna que je n'ai pas assez loué tant pour sa beauté forte que pour sa complaisance nous a bien soignés. Il y a du sel. Le vin est bon. Mais pendant qu'on mange, on file. Tetuan n'est plus là, non plus que la tour Martin ; nous voilà sous une immense muraille de rochers à pic – arrêtons nous dans une fente de rochers ; nous serons au calme et plus confortablement pour déjeuner. Car bien que la mer soit calme : le sol du bateau est peu stable pendant sa marche. Nous voilà donc blottis dans un coin, comme des corsaires barbaresques du bon vieux temps prêts à faire quelque mauvais coup. Le rocher est sombre, l'eau sous le bateau est tellement claire et transparente qu'on y voie à des profondeurs énormes – par ci par là quelques pingouins ? au long bec font leur métier de chasseurs ; un gros poisson épineux rouge et jaune se présente à la surface de l'eau où il flotte ; il est malade ou blessé ; on l'amène. Il est temps de partir. Tout le monde est satisfait. [**14-d**] Le vent souffle ferme : le bateau est frappé par l'eau qui retourne sur nous en pluie épaisse ; on s'enveloppe et l'on se tasse, on arrivera quelque peu mouillé peu importe, tout va bien – mais voilà le vent qui tombe ; il faut la rame. Décidément nous n'arriverons pas en 3 heures. De fait il est déjà nuit quand nous approchons de la pêcherie ; mais les lumières de la maison de Bajonna sont en vue : un quart d'heure après on nous aide à sortir du bateau – adieu, à demain – et nous reprenons le chemin de la fonda ; où après avoir diné, nous nous couchons.

14 août – le lendemain matin il faut être prêt de bonne heure. Le bateau de Ceuta part à 7 heures. Nous descendons la grande rue qui conduit au port – une fois de plus nous retrouvons les maures et les juifs qui à Ceuta forment peut-être un bon tiers de la population.

Bajonna nous accompagne jusque [**15-a**] au bateau. Aaron le juif nous quitte d'un air mélancolique. Le pourboire lui a-t-il paru insuffisant ? Il était honorable cependant. Il se consolera.

Adieu. Le bateau part. Nous serons dans 3 heures à Algesiras. La mer est tranquille comme Baptiste dans le détroit. Je regarde Ceuta s'éloigner. Le môle, la ville sur la presqu'ile qui rattache ce dernier au Maroc. Dans Ceuta il y a 3 ou 4 palmiers. il n'y en avait pas un seul à Tetuan ou les alentours – Je revois le vieux Ceuta, la caserne fort, les tours espagnols juchées sur les pitons de la frontière – derrière la vallée sombre qui sépare du Maroc les possessions Espagnoles – adieu ou au revoir ...qui sait ?

Le temps passe : nous tournons maintenant les yeux du côté Europe : voilà Gibraltar voilà Algesiras. Peu à peu la ville se dessine : voici le port où est Burty [**15-b**] est ce petit point noir que l'on voit là-bas sur la jetée – cela grandit, grandit grossit et atteint bientôt la grosseur naturelle qui comme vous le savez n'est pas mince. C'est lui...Il est là, tristement, tout seul ...oui tout seul...son mauvais ange l'a lâchement abandonné après lui avoir fait faire le coup.

Donc notre pauvre ami, par suite d'une fâcheuse suggestion venue d'un consul hypochondriaque est resté huit jours à se morfondre dans une triste ville de province, tandis que nous autres nous revenons chargés de souvenirs charmants et ineffaçables – Voilà ce que c'est mon ami que de s'arrêter aux bagatelles de la porte...oui je le sais bien...quand nous sommes partis le vent était *d'est*, Gibraltar avait *son chapeau* – la mer était un peu houleuse :... mais à tout prendre notre petit voyage d'Afrique [15-c] valait bien 2 heures de mal de mer, qui peut-être ne serait pas venue – et quand vous allez en Angleterre vous n'y regardez pas de si près.

Donc vous êtes impardonnable : aussi êtes-vous un peu pâle et un peu défait : assez piètre mine malgré la belle cravate bleue à points blancs que vous avez achetée, pour vous faire bien venir dans les guilledous d'Algesiras – ah poète!! Trois fois poète, quelle leçon!! Et comment allez vous vous tirer de là quand on vous demandera des nouvelles d'Afrique. Car il ne faut pas plaider le cas de maladie devant des médecins – il ne vous reste plus qu'à vous armer contre l'ironie O Scipion l'africain, Oh. Comte d'Algesiras y Tetuan!!!!. Voilà ce que c'est que de se laisser terrifier par *le chapeau de Gibraltar*!

Demain nous nous embarquerons à Gibraltar pour Malaga. Et de Malaga nous irons à Grenade rendre à la mère la visite promise. [15-d] aller visiter Grendade après Tetuan c'est, en effet logique. On dit qu'à Tetuan bien des gens gardent la clef de leur maison de Grenade avec l'espoir d'y revenir un jour. Quand l'ambassadeur du Maroc m'a-t-on dit a visité l'Espagne, dans Cordoue, Tolède il est resté impassible ; mais à Grenade, dans l'alhambra il a été pris d'une émotion qu'il n'a pu cacher. Il a demandé qu'on s'éloignât un instant et il s'est mis à pleurer toutes ses larmes!!!! – les assistants pleurèrent aussi.

C'est que Tetuan c'est Grenade et Grenade c'est Tetuan. D'ailleurs Grenade c'est encore une ville maure ; l'indolence des habitants, leur amour du laissez faire, tout rappelle encore la domination maure de telle sorte que quand on a vu Tetuan et que du haut du Généralife on regarde Grenade il n'est pas difficile avec un petit effort de vision interne de reconstituer la Grenade du 15e siècle.

IV

Select Bibliography

(see notes for further sources)

Berchet, Jean-Claude, *Le voyage en Orient* (Paris: Robert Laffont, 1985).

Bessis, Henriette, "Philippe Burty et Eugène Delacroix," *Gazette des Beaux-Arts* 72 (1968): 195–202.

Bonduelle, Michel, "Charcot et l'Italie," *Neurologia Psichiatria Scienze Umane*, 17 (1997): 179–89.

Burty, Philippe "Eugène Delacroix au Maroc," *Gazette des Beaux-Arts* 19 (1865): 144–154.

Charcot, Jean-Martin, "Banquet offert à M. le professeur Charcot," *Le Progrès Médical* (1883, 8 décembre): 999–1001.

_____ *Leçons du mardi à la Salpêtrière: Policlinique 1887–88, 1888–89*, 2 vols. (Paris: Progrès Médical, 1887, 1889, 1892).

_____ and Paul Richer, *Les démoniaques dans l'art* (Paris: Delahaye et Lecrosnier, 1887).

_____ and Paul Richer, *Les difformes et les malades dans l'art* (Paris: Lecrosnier et Babe, 1889).

Delacroix, Eugène, *Correspondance*, ed. Philippe Burty (Paris 1880) vol. 1.

_____ *Journal*, ed. Paul Flat et René Piot, t. 1 (1823–1850), (Paris: Plon, 1893).

_____ "Une Noce Juive dans le Maroc," *Magasin Pittoresque* 10 (1842): 28–30.

_____ *Souvenirs d'un voyage dans le Maroc*, édition de Laure Beaumont-Maillet, Barthélémy Jobert et Sophie Join-Lambert (Paris: Gallimard, 1999).

Didier, Charles, " Le Maroc," *Revue des Deux Mondes*, (1836, 8 novembre): 241–269.

Freud, Sigmund, "Charcot," in *The Standard Edition of the Complete Psychological Works*, trans. and ed. by James Strachey (London: The Hogarth Press, 1966–74), vol. 3, 11–23.

_____ *On the History of the Psycho-analytic Movement* (1914) in *The Standard Edition of the Complete Psychological Works*, vol. 14, 7–66.

Gelfand, Toby, "'Mon cher docteur Freud': Charcot's unpublished correspondence to Freud, 1888–1893." *Bulletin of the History of Medicine* 62 (1988): 563–588.

_____ "Charcot's response to Freud's rebellion," *Journal of the History of Ideas* 50 (1989): 293–307.

_____ "From Religious to Bio-Medical Anti-Semitism: The Career of Jules Soury" in *French Medical Culture in the Nineteenth Century*, ed. A. La Berge and M. Feingold, (Rodopi:Amsterdam and Atlanta, 1994): 248–279.

_____ "Charcot's Brains," *Brain and Language*, 69 (1999): 31–55.

Gilman, Sander L., "Jews and Mental Illness: Medical Metaphors, Anti-Semitism, and the Jewish Response," *Journal of the History of the Behavioral Sciences* 20 (1984): 150–159. Reprinted as "The Madness of the Jews," in Gilman, *Difference and Pathology. Stereotypes of Sexuality, Race and Madness*, (Ithaca and London: Cornell University Press, 1985): 150–162.

Goetz, Christopher G, Michel Bonduelle, and Toby Gelfand, *Charcot: Constructing Neurology* (New York: Oxford University Press, 1995).

Goldstein, Jan, "The Wandering Jew and the Problem of Psychiatric Anti-semitism in Fin-de-Siècle France," *Journal of Contemporary History*, 20 (1985): 521–552.

Jobert, Barthélémy, *Delacroix* (Paris: Gallimard, 1997).

Kalman, Julie, "Sensuality, Depravity, and Ritual Murder: The Damascus Blood Libel and Jews in France, *Jewish Social Studies* 13 (2007): 35–58.

Meige, Henry, *Étude sur certains Névropathes Voyageurs. Le Juif errant à la Salpêtrière* (Paris, thesis, 1893),

———— "Charcot Artiste," *Nouvelle Iconographie de la Salpêtrière* 11 (1898): 489–516.

Miège, Jean-Louis, *Le Maroc et l'Europe (1830–1894)*, (Paris: Presses Universitaires de France, 1963), vol. 4.

Mirbeau, Octave, "Le siècle de Charcot" in *Chroniques du diable*, ed. Pierre Michel, (*Annales littéraires de l'Université de Besançon*, 555, Diffusion les Belles Lettres: Paris, 1995):121–127.

Paléologue, Maurice, "Le Maroc. Notes et Souvenirs," *Revue des Deux Mondes* 83 (1885,15 avril): 888–924.

Séailles, Gaston, *A Dehodencqu*, 2 ed., (Paris: Société de Propagation des livres d'art, 1910).

Sergines, "Les échos de Paris," *Les Annales politiques et littéraires* 21 (1893, 27 août): 133.

Silverman, Deborah, *Art Nouveau in Fin-de-Siècle France* (Berkeley: University of California Press, 1989).

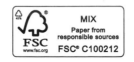

Printed in February 2012
by Gauvin Press,
Gatineau, Québec